Skinny Chick!

The Secret Formula for Losing Fat
Quickly Without Ever Being Hungry

Robin Webb

Published by Best Seller Publishing®, Pasadena, CA
Best Seller Publishing® is a registered trademark
Printed in the United States of America.

This publication is designed to provide accurate and authoritative information with regard to the subject matter covered. It is sold with the understanding that the publisher is not engaged in rendering legal, accounting, or other professional advice. If legal advice or other expert assistance is required, the services of a competent professional should be sought. The opinions expressed by the authors in this book are not endorsed by Best Seller Publishing® and are the sole responsibility of the author rendering the opinion.

Most Best Seller Publishing® titles are available at special quantity discounts for bulk purchases for sales promotions, premiums, fundraising, and educational use. Special versions or book excerpts can also be created to fit specific needs.

For more information, please write:
Best Seller Publishing®
1346 Walnut Street, #205
Pasadena, CA 91106
or call 1(626) 765 9750
Toll Free: 1(844) 850-3500
Visit us online at: www.BestSellerPublishing.org

Table of Contents

Dedication

This book is dedicated to the love of my life, my husband Chris, who always supports and believes in me; even when I have a hard time believing in myself. To my mom who was the first person to show me what unconditional love is: and to my little sunshine, Alyssa who gives me a reason to always want to be a better person, teaches me so much and brings so much joy to my life.

Introduction

"Nothing worth having was ever achieved
without effort."

Theodore Roosevelt

I am so thrilled that you decided to read my labor of love, *Skinny Chick*! I have watched so many people transform their bodies and lives using my system and it brings me great joy that you will now join the many that have already discovered that you can take charge of your body and health! Weight loss... has any subject been more overdone? I get it... you have tried everything. Some things worked in the beginning and then stopped working; some things worked but as soon as you stopped, you gained all the weight back. One thing I get from almost every client I encounter is this, I hate dieting! I hear you... so do I! So what makes my program different from all of the other programs you have tried and failed with? Simple, I am not interested in simply helping you lose weight. I am interested in helping you lose weight while forever changing your relationship with food so this will be the last weight loss plan you ever do!

Losing weight the typical calories in versus calories out way makes you lose a lot of muscle mass and water weight but does not do much to your actual fat stores. This is why you lose twenty pounds but still feel squishy and do not like your shape. Fat is not a heavy thing; muscle actually weighs twice as much as fat. So imagine what losing five pounds of fat (fluff) versus five pounds of muscle will do for you… getting a nice mental picture. One of the MANY benefits you can expect to glean from my program is to lose 97% pure fat or more if you do it correctly. Not only that, you will lose it more quickly than you ever thought possible!

You can expect to lose up to five to seven pounds in the first week and up to three pounds of pure fat a week after that! I have many clients who lose weight significantly faster than that, and I have clients who don't lose quite that fast. My clients all have one thing in common though: they all lose fat on this plan if they do it consistently and in the way I have it laid out… even the clients who have tried everything else and it hasn't worked.

Another big factor for so many of my clients is that they can't stop craving junk food so they do well for a while with other programs and then fall of the wagon. This program is designed to heal your metabolic issues and end your cravings. Can you imagine not craving sugar anymore? Can you imagine wanting healthy food and liking how it tastes? It can be a reality for you just like it is for me and so many of my fantastic clients. All of this can be done without starving yourself! In fact, you won't be hungry. It is very typical for clients to tell me they have to force themselves to eat sometimes because they are simply not hungry while on my program. The other thing that makes this program different from any other program is this: I will not leave you hanging once you are done with the rapid fat loss portion. I will teach you a real, doable way to eat for life that is not restricted all the time; in fact, I am a believer in treating yourself!

I am also a firm believer in the fact that most people would have a healthier lifestyle if they knew what constituted a healthy diet and had a way to achieve that. How can one eat only healthy food though when they constantly have strong cravings for unhealthy food? The simple answer is they can't. Very few people have such strong will power; I certainly did not before I figured out the secrets. The other issue my fabulous clients have is they want to lose weight but they have worked really, really hard and they still don't get where they really want to be with their weight loss goals (I have been there!). This causes them to have an 'oh well then I quit, I can't get there attitude.'

When my clients get desperate enough to find me, they are so happy and grateful to have something that works! In fact, they tend to get "greedy": 'I only lost 2% body fat this week?! That sucks… I'm not happy.' I have to remind them, 'Have you ever lost that much in a week before, let alone all fat?' 'Well, no.' Okay then, cut yourself some slack!

My favorite clients are the ones who have tried everything because they truly appreciate how well this works and finally feel free from their weight issues for good. Don't get me wrong, I love all of my clients but my least favorite ones are the ones who are on a program for the first time ever and it happens to be mine. They often do not appreciate how well this works and how different it is because they simply have nothing to compare it to.

This book is the key to finally unlock the health and vibrance you have inside you that is just waiting to be released. If you do the work, you can attain the body you want, have vibrant health, unlimited energy, and banish your cravings and desire to gorge yourself with unhealthy food for good. There is just one catch... you actually have to do it.

Are you ready to finally live this one life in the body you really desire? Surrender yourself to this journey of discovering that body… you will not regret it. Take your power and control back!

I like to share my story of what lead me to the world of health and nutrition and why I know without a doubt that you CAN change your body no matter where you are in your journey. I began to have a lot of health issues in my early twenties. By my early to mid-twenties, I had gall bladder issues, liver issues, Crohn's disease, fertility issues, hypothyroid issues, Candida overgrowth, and so many other small things in between. I also struggled with my weight, although it was hard to see it on me because I have a very small frame. I was essentially a "skinny fat person" and I had a lot of weight and inflammation around my middle. I was obviously very unhealthy and completely miserable. I vividly remember lying in bed and contemplating ending my life and how I would do it… no, I am not exaggerating, that is how much pain and misery I was in. I also remember hoping and wishing for a cure to my multitude of health issues.

In the course of about two years, I went to specialist after specialist trying to figure out what was so wrong with me and why despite the best care, I kept getting worse! In the beginning, nobody ever tried to really figure out why I was so sick; they just kept giving me drug after drug after drug to try. Some medication would help for a little while and then stop helping; some made me worse. I always ended up right back where I started and often with a new health issue. My lowest point came when I had a near fatal and severe reaction to one of my many medications. I heard my doctor tell the person I was with at the time that he did not know if I would make it through the night. I remember thinking: 'Maybe this is the answer then.' I was so exhausted from being sick and miserable that I just completely gave up.

However, I have always been very stubborn at heart. At some point throughout the night of my near-death experience, something came over me. I decided that not only would I make it, I would be healthy. I did not know how but I knew I would! I was no longer content with just surviving and hoping for a cure... I wanted to thrive. My doctors recommended that I remove the majority of my colon, my gallbladder, and give up on the notion of ever having children. At first, this news was devastating. I tried very hard to picture my life this way and accept my fate, and I ultimately became very depressed.

As I said before though, my stubborn spirit would not allow that. I had already started down the path to a healthier lifestyle with juicing and cutting out gluten and it had already helped me a bit. Why not get REALLY into this health stuff and see if it made me all the way better? What on earth did I have to lose at this point? I decided that I was not having multiple organs removed or taking any more drugs, and I immersed myself into healthy eating, detoxification, meditation, exercise, supplements, etc., etc. No matter how crazy or far-fetched it seemed, I would try it. I had decided I would thrive and I was going to do anything it took to make that happen.

Let me paint a picture of how my life looked before this. Fast food... every day at least one meal if not more. Family sized bags of M&Ms... consumed in one night by only me and often. Bottles of wine in one night... again consumed by me alone. I don't even know how much booze... oh and I smoked. Then I would go on crash/starvation diets in between but I really had no clue what constituted healthy eating.

Let me tell you, going from a lifestyle that looks like that to a very healthy lifestyle all of a sudden... not easy or pretty! I tried many things that did not work. I fell on my face and fell off the wagon so many times, but I would get back up, dust myself off, carry on, and keep trying. I had the picture of what I wanted in my mind and I held onto that.

Today I can proudly say, I got to the vision in my head. I have all of my organs and they work great. I have a healthy little seven-year-old girl and at the writing of this book, I am actually pregnant with my second little girl. I am fitter than I have ever been in my adult life. I do not have symptoms of Crohn's disease, hypothyroidism, gallbladder disease, Candida overgrowth, or any of the other things that ruined my life back then. I do however have a ton of energy and a body that supports me. Would you like that too? I am offering you a place to start, a blueprint. You just have to do it, that is all, just do it! If I can overcome everything I did, you can too.

You have already taken the first step in deciding to buy my book… are you ready to leave the body that does not support you, that you are not proud of behind? Are you ready to step into the body you want? No matter how many times you have failed before, you can do this! Dedicate yourself to doing this program with discipline and follow it to the letter, and you WILL get results!

My intention in writing this book was to spread health and wellness as far and as wide as I possibly can. After my horrible health issues and near-death experience followed by my healing and new lease on life, I decided that my mission in life was to spread this knowledge to others. I have a little nutrition clinic called Complete Weight Loss and Wellness in Denver, CO where I have seen and continue to see many clients and have helped them transform their lives for the better. Although I do love consulting, my time is limited and I can only reach so many people this way. That is why I decided to write a book. I had no idea how I would do anything with this book but as soon as I set my intention on getting this information out there; it all fell into place pretty effortlessly.

I have a funny story though. Weight loss was not what I set out to specialize in. Nope, it was digestive health, diabetes, cancer, etc. I remember being at a party and having a guy ask me about my studies while I was in school to earn my degree in nutrition. He said, 'So you learn about the food pyramid and weight loss and stuff right?' At that time, I had completely turned my own life around by changing my lifestyle and it was a hard road! I found his assumption that nutritionists just learn the food pyramid and weight loss and stuff insulting (in hindsight it was obviously not meant to insult me).

It was not until I gained sixty-five pounds while I was pregnant with my first daughter and had the enormous challenge of losing all that weight did I realize how complicated and not straightforward weight loss actually is. I figured out very quickly that starving yourself does not work because that just makes you binge later and that most people just can't maintain it (not to mention how unhealthy it is).

The calories in versus calories out thing… no, not really that helpful. I worked out like crazy; the weight just would not budge. The weight I did lose was not primarily fat and I would still feel squishy no matter how low I got my weight. I got myself down to a little below my ideal weight and I still had a squishy gut and thighs! It forced me to look harder and figure out why I, like so many women, could not get very far with these futile methods.

What lies in this book is some of the tricks I have learned over the years. One thing I love about what I do now: it is not JUST weight loss (not that there is anything wrong with *just* doing weight loss), there is so much more to it. I always say that I discovered a weight loss plan that can secretly and cleverly act as detoxification, body healing, and so much more.

One of the best outcomes of my years in practice with clients is all the other benefits my lovely clients gained by teaching them my way of life. I also realize after my own struggle with weight loss how very disheartening it is to try so hard to get that weight off and to have it not budge, come off so slowly, or still be squishy. How much it hurt my self-esteem when my friend's daughter asked me if I was pregnant again… a year after I had my baby! How I hated shopping for clothing because nothing fit and I did not like how I looked. How I started to be sucked into the black hole of, 'Maybe I have to accept my body this way, maybe this is just who I am now.' I looked in the mirror and hated what I saw. Yes, I have experienced all of these things, just as you likely have. Please whole-heartedly try this blue print to escape it and free yourself from it for good! You do not have to accept not liking your body.

I would like to take the opportunity to point out that I am not against modern medicine. On the contrary, I am fascinated by it. I am humbled and amazed by all of the advances in science that greater minds than mine have brought to us and the ways it can enrich and save human lives. My big issue with it is this: we can't expect to treat our bodies horribly and then take a magic pill to fix it when our unhealthy lifestyle causes it to fall apart and stop working the way it should. We need to treat our bodies, our temples, and the only home we have to live in, with the care and respect it deserves if we expect it to treat us well back. If we need medicine, surgery, or whatever else along the way, fine! Thank goodness we have the option! This does not mean we should carelessly abuse our bodies to the point of forcing ourselves to need these interventions.

I also have a deep respect for the doctors and nurses in the medical profession. Please do not take anything I am saying as a reason to ignore the advice of your doctor or discount modern medicine. If it is used properly, I think it is useful and often necessary. It is also important to listen to yourself. If something does not resonate with you, regardless of who it is coming from, pay attention to that. Most importantly, take good care of the one body you have so your checkups with your doctor can just be to find out that all is well!

While we are at it, let me list the people who should not under any circumstances do the Skinny Chick! Rapid Fat Loss portion of this plan. Pregnant women, do not do any rapid weight loss protocol while pregnant. You can eat as if you were on maintenance but while pregnant is not the time to try to lose weight in such a drastic way. If you are breastfeeding, you will drastically cut down your milk supply. Again, eat sensibly and eat as if on maintenance. You can do the Rapid Fat Loss portion when you are done nursing. If you have or have ever had kidney disease, I strongly recommend you don't do the Skinny Chick! Rapid Fat Loss portion, as it can overtax your kidneys for those whose kidneys are already overtaxed (that will make more sense as you get further into reading about the program). At the very least get the okay from your doctor and have your doctor monitor you. If you are taking medication for blood pressure, heart disease, or diabetes, you will need to be monitored by your doctor while on this program.

It is possible for people to drastically cut their doses back on their medications with proper diet and lifestyle changes and even stop taking them completely, which is great. While in the process however, if you are taking the wrong dosage of medication, you can have some seriously unpleasant side effects (such as blood pressure getting too low and blood sugar issues). If you are on any medication for any serious illness, consult with your doctor to be safe. If you have hypothyroidism like I do, you will need to do this in a different way. This is outlined at the beginning of Chapter 3, so you don't end up lowering your levels and feeling terrible. If you have hypothyroidism, do not do the rapid loss portion unless your condition is well under control with medication. With hypothyroidism, you can also expect it to work a little more slowly. That is not always the case for everybody, I know for me it is. I am a nutritionist, not a doctor, I do not have a medical degree so if you are unsure if it is unsafe in any way to lose weight so quickly, consult with your doctor.

It is just food but I take the safety of my clients very, very seriously so please pay attention to your body and seek help if you feel you need it. One more warning, if you are on birth control (pill or shot form), there is a hypothetical risk that it will not be as effective while you are in the Rapid Fat Loss phase. I strongly recommend a backup method as even a hypothetical risk is not worth it if a pregnancy is not wanted.

"How does one become a butterfly? They have to want to learn to fly so much that they are willing to give up being a caterpillar."

Trina Paulus

Chapter 1
Weight Loss, Why is it so Difficult?

Ah nutrition and diets... a much debated, sometimes very controversial subject. Why does everybody have such different opinions? Because there is so much information out there, it can make your head spin! In addition, it changes constantly. Eggs and butter used to cause heart disease... now they are healthy. High carb, low fat... no wait... low carb, high protein... what gives?! I have to be honest here: everything I am saying is also simply my opinion. My opinion is based on a ravenous and obsessive hunger for researching, reading, and absorbing everything I can get my hands on about nutrition and health and then trying out my theories. So it is not baseless... but my opinion nonetheless. The reason I bring this up is that you will need to listen to your body along the way. If something does not work well in your body, don't do it, no matter who tells you to. Remember, you are the only true expert on yourself.

With that being said… what do you think your body turns into the fat stored in your fat cells? Did you say fat? You would be wrong! It is actually excess carbohydrates that your body turns into fat. Let's go through a very simplistic crash course on how your body stores fat.

Let's examine how our body creates energy from food. Your body uses three primary sources for energy in the following order: glucose (carbohydrates), protein, and then fat. Our bodies prefer carbohydrates, as this is the easiest source of energy. The body can use protein if it needs to but it actually needs carbohydrates, so protein and no carbohydrates is not an answer to weight loss. Fat (as in fat from our fat cells) is only used as energy if there is no other option.

Does your body ever not have access to carbohydrates and protein? Probably not. Our early ancestors lived in a world of feast or famine. There were times when they would have plenty to eat so they would eat a lot and would try to pack pounds on (imagine that). There were times when there was no food so they would have to live off this energy stored as the fat in their fat cells. We have evolved past these early people in so many ways. For most people, food is now abundant and available at any time. However, one way we did not evolve is that our body still stores the excess fat for the next time it needs to use the stored energy or fat from the fat cells in a time of famine.

Back to the question: how do we store fat? As I said above, your body turns excess carbohydrates into fat. Any carbohydrate you eat that is not immediately used for energy is stored in the fat cells. Let's take the example of a simple carbohydrate and a complex carbohydrate. A simple carbohydrate is one that has been broken down by a lot of processing, such as table sugar or white flour. A complex carbohydrate is one that has not been broken down, such as a whole grain like brown rice. Simple carbohydrates are very easy for the body to digest, which means that they go into the bloodstream to be used by the cells as energy very easily and quickly. Complex carbohydrates require some work for the body to break down or digest so they go into the blood stream to be used by cells as energy at a much slower rate.

Here is a visual for you of what happens when you eat a carbohydrate, your body's preferred energy source. We will use the example of a candy bar and a very whole grain brown rice (minimally processed takes forty-five plus minutes to cook). Example one: you eat your very whole grain brown rice. Your body will break down or digest the rice to its simplest form, glucose (what your cells actually use for energy), at about the rate of twenty five or so calories per minute, releasing a steady stream of glucose into your blood stream. When glucose hits your bloodstream, your pancreas responds by releasing insulin. The insulin is the catalyst to get the glucose into your cells to use as energy. When the cells have their immediate needs met (if you are sitting on the couch watching TV, their needs will be met very quickly), there will likely be glucose leftover in the blood stream. We can't have glucose in the bloodstream, so the body will do what it needs to do to get the glucose out of the bloodstream. The body will take whatever the cells do not have immediate use for and put it in your fat cells for storage.

Now let's examine what happens when you eat a candy bar that is chock full of simple sugar. Your body will break this carbohydrate into its simplest form of glucose at the rate of about one hundred calories per minute, causing a rush of glucose into your blood stream. Your pancreas will do what it is supposed to do and release insulin in kind. With the rush of the sugar, there will be a matching rush of insulin. As with the glucose from the brown rice, which is exactly the same as far as your cells are concerned, your cells will get their glucose needs met and then take the rest and store it in the fat cells. However, as glucose keeps rushing into your blood stream, your body keeps frantically producing insulin, leading to an over-production of insulin. Your body will frantically try to take all of the extra glucose out of your blood stream and put it in your fat cells, and, of course, it will eventually succeed. When the insulin is all done with that, there will be a lot of excess insulin in your blood stream.

Any excess insulin must be removed from the blood stream and sent to the kidneys to be excreted. With the first example, where there is just a little insulin left in the blood stream after it has completed its task of removing all glucose from the blood stream, your body will clear it out pretty easily. With the second example of too much insulin being put into the blood stream, there will be a severe excess of leftover insulin after all the glucose has been removed from the bloodstream. Our bodies can only get rid of the excess insulin so fast, so several things happen from there which we will get to in a minute.

A person with type 1 diabetes will tell you that insulin is unbelievably important. After all, without it, one can't get glucose into their cells. Type 1 diabetes is when one can't produce insulin or can't produce enough and has to inject it so that they can get glucose into their cells. People are typically born with it.

Type 2 diabetes is just the opposite. A person with type 2 diabetes has chronically too much insulin in their blood stream so their cells become ambivalent toward it and no longer respond to insulin; thus, not getting glucose into the cells. People typically develop it later in life due to an unhealthy lifestyle. As a matter of fact, type 2 diabetes used to be called Adult Onset Diabetes but was changed to type 2 diabetes due to the fact that so many younger people started getting it. It is my belief that food can not only prevent this ailment but also heal it. It actually irritates me to no end to hear that we need to find a cure when the prevention and the reversal of it are the same in most cases.

Remember all the insulin left over in your blood stream after you ate that candy bar? It will sit there and saturate your cells as I said above while it is waiting to be pushed out of the blood stream and into the kidneys. Over time, the cells get so used to being bathed in insulin that they don't respond to it anymore (insulin no longer acts as the catalyst to push glucose into the cells). This is a very simplistic explanation of type 2 diabetes but basically, the cells no longer respond to insulin.

There is more though. The insulin also gets "bored" while it waits to be excreted and calls for more carbohydrates to be consumed to occupy it. Unfortunately, the excess insulin in your system will not communicate with the pancreas so the pancreas will not know there is already insulin in the system and therefore, it will pump out more insulin. Do you see where this is going? I call this cycle the sugar roller coaster.

Have you noticed when you have a sugary cereal and orange juice for breakfast, you are starving around two hours or so later? This is why, when you start your day like that, you are setting yourself up to ride the sugar roller coaster all day long. Over time, aside from the fact that you are setting your cells up not to uptake glucose properly (which will make your body think it needs more), you are also setting your pancreas up to overreact every time you consume anything with glucose in it.

The excess insulin has also been shown to lead to other things such as heart disease, mood swings, hormone issues, and a myriad of other issues well beyond the scope of this book or my expertise. Years and years of doing this to your body will eventually lead to insulin resistance or what has been dubbed syndrome X (pre-diabetic) and ultimately type 2 diabetes. If you already have type 2 diabetes, this diet can help you regain some insulin sensitivity, helping you with your pancreas. It, however, does take time to achieve this if your body is already to this stage. If you are on the verge of type 2 diabetes, this diet might help you reverse that more quickly. The best case scenario is to always limit this kind of food so you never need to reverse it. It is much easier to prevent disease than reverse it. An ounce of prevention is worth a pound of cure.

So what can you do? How can you get off this sugar roller coaster if you keep craving sugar? This is where the Skinny Chick! Rapid Fat Loss portion of this plan comes into play. This plan does several things to reverse all of the above.

First, it takes simple carbohydrates out of the picture (don't panic, your body will stop wanting them). What we will be doing is tricking your body into bypassing its need to use carbohydrates as energy and start using your fat cells as energy. This eliminates the storage of excess carbohydrates, while emptying your fat cells and using the contents as its energy source. This concept is not new... it is called ketosis. I have found a way to do it so that it works more quickly and in a very safe and healthy way. You need to know that you will be getting a lot of calories from your fat stores that your body has been saving for the famine that never comes. These extra calories from your fat cells are part of the reason you can be on a diet and not be hungry. Will it still take some willpower? Yes, it will! You have likely spent years and years setting your body up for metabolic disorders with bad habits. The aim of this program is not only to help you get rid of the byproducts of those bad habits (stored fat and toxicity). It is also to teach yourself new, more healthy habits and to get your body to a point where you are not constantly craving this unhealthy food so you can stop feeding the sugar monster.

Second, this program lets your pancreas have a break so it can heal and not continue to overact to carbohydrates. Your cells will also get this break so they can eventually become more sensitive to insulin again. This is part of the piece of not gaining the weight back. Getting into the concept and complexity of self-healing is well beyond the scope of this book but I will use an example to demonstrate my point. Our bodies have an innate ability to heal themselves. Think about when you get a cut; do you need to do anything to heal your cut aside from ensuring it does not get infected? No, your body regenerates itself and heals your broken skin with no intervention whatsoever from you. The rest of our body can do this too. The issue is, if parts of your body, such as your pancreas, continue to get pounded down, causing it to break down; it never gets the opportunity to heal. Think again of the cut: if you keep picking at it, does it heal? You need to leave it alone and not intervene to let it heal. You will be giving your pancreas the opportunity to be left alone and heal during the three-week Skinny Chick! Rapid Fat Loss portion and beyond.

When you resume eating more carbohydrates in the maintenance part of the program, (I will teach you how to do this without causing your pancreas to get to this state again), your pancreas won't overact. This also derails you from the sugar roller coaster. If you have abused your body your entire life, keep in mind that it may take you more than three weeks to re-set your pancreas and eliminate cravings. How long it takes to heal depends on how devoted you are to sticking to the program and what shape your body is in when you start out. I know that the discovery of the concept of letting the body heal naturally was life changing for me. I hope you will give it a chance so it can be for you too. If you just give your body a break by not filling it with unhealthy and toxic things, it will heal and regenerate itself.

Third, it will detoxify you. Toxicity is yet another thing standing in the way of weight loss. Our bodies have a beautiful detoxification system that works very hard to clear all of the junk out of your body. Think of your detoxification system as the garbage man of your body. Our early ancestors were not exposed to many toxins. They ate the food they caught and gathered or grew, and there was no such thing as artificial colorings, preservatives, pesticides, etc... etc. This is another area in which our bodies have not evolved: our bodies are so inundated with toxins that in many cases, it can't clear them all out of our systems. The trash man in our body has to do something with all of this trash. Just like glucose, our body would prefer it if the toxins were not floating around in our blood stream. So, it starts finding places to store them. Here enters the fat cell. The garbage man in the body trying to figure out what to do with all of these toxins it can't get through the already overwhelmed elimination system sees this closet (the fat cell) sitting there, not being used. The fat cells are filled with a protective layer of goo (the fat inside the fat cell) that will keep the "biohazardous waste" (a little dramatic perhaps) safely inside. Perfect! The excess can be stored in there! This is what our bodies do with all those toxins it can't clear out fast enough. Fat cells are biologically inactive... the only purpose they serve is to store calories in case they are needed for famine and insulation (which we do need some of). So our body puts the toxins in there until it can get to dealing with them, which it never gets to. How likely do you think your body is going to be to open up those closets and dump those toxins out into your blood stream... not likely! Our bodies are interested in survival, not dumping toxins into the blood stream. This is one of the ways so many diets fall short and fail. Eating a diet full of artificial preservatives, artificial colors, artificial sweeteners, and so on that your body does not know what to do with and sees as a toxin furthers the toxic load on your body. If your body already has a lot of toxins to deal with, it is not going to dump the contents of your fat cells, which are very toxic, into your blood stream to get rid of them. This is one of the many reasons you end up losing water and muscle mass as opposed to fat on many diets. Your body needs to deal with what you are putting in it first! With primarily whole food in the Skinny Chick! Rapid Fat Loss system, you won't be putting junk into your body. Your body will take this opportunity to dump the stored up junk that it has in its closets. The goo lining the closets flushes out too, freeing you from your built up fat stores, along with the toxic gunk you don't want in your body. The food choices on the diet are also selected to give you a combination of good flavor and healthy foods that will aid your body in getting rid of the toxins and the stored fat.

Fourth, the plan keeps your body from getting over-acidic. While in ketosis, your body is undergoing a complicated biological process as it breaks down your fat cells to use as energy. Instead of using glucose for energy, your body will be using ketones, the byproduct of this process. Ketones are very acidic by nature, as is the toxic material stored in your fat cells so if you are adding more acidity to the mix through not eating the right things (almost all junk food and highly processed food is highly acidic), your weight loss will slow to a screeching halt. The reason for this, in part, is that our bodies have to keep a certain pH balance to survive. If there is excess acidity in your body, your body will be very preoccupied with getting that acidity level back down to normal and will not be interested in dumping out the content of your fat cells. This will only add MORE acidity. The food choices for this diet were chosen in part for their alkalizing effect, meaning the acidity in your body stays normal or perhaps becomes normal for the first time, allowing your body to focus on dumping fat and healing instead of trying to keep its pH level normal. On many diet plans, there is a large selection of foods made out of chemicals, artificial colors, preservatives, and artificial sweeteners. First, this kind of food does NOT taste good. Second, do you have a better understanding as to why these nutrient negative foods (I will explain nutrient negative foods in chapter 4 of this book) may actually slow your weight loss down? From a business standpoint, this model is smart. If people need to continue to buy their chemical diet food to continue to pursue weight loss, they have a customer for a very long time, if not for life! I understand business and I know that teaching my clients to eat healthily with real food so they are not dependent on me for the rest of their life is not the most brilliant business model. The aim of my program is to teach you to be able to do this on your own nonetheless as this is how you can *really* keep your new, slimmer figure for the rest of your life.

Fifth, you will be eating primarily whole foods in a way that tastes good. Over time, your body will start wanting more and more of this food, and it will stop wanting all the junk you were eating before. Your taste buds will start working better and become more sensitive, and super sweet or super salty foods will taste terrible to you (cake frosting or anything super sweet literally makes me gag now…it didn't in the past). I will explain this in more detail in the maintenance phase chapter (chapter 4) that you will undertake after you get to your goal weight and in between weeks when you are not on the Skinny Chick! Rapid Fat Loss Protocol.

A quote from a client after her first three weeks on the rapid weight loss portion: 'I never realized cauliflower was so sweet!' Can you imagine cauliflower tasting sweet to you? How much would your life change for the better if that happened to you? I don't want you to just lose weight, I want you to change your habits and change your life. I want you to be free of your struggle FOREVER! One of the reasons my clients are so successful on my plan is that by simply resetting your body chemistry, so that as time goes by it takes less and less willpower, added to the fact that you will see results, creates a person who can and will stick with it until they get to their goal! Trust me when I say, once you reset your insulin resistance issues and get to your goal weight, maintaining it is so much easier than losing it. Meaning you can get away with treats without blowing your diet or gaining weight. I will teach you how in the maintenance chapter.

"Don't trade what you want in this moment for what you want for your future."

Author Unknown

Chapter 2
Skinny Chick! Rapid Fat Loss Protocol

Now let's start melting off your excess fat! Read this book very thoroughly before beginning your program, as it is imperative this is done correctly. If not done correctly, you will feel terrible and will very likely quit before you start to see your amazing results. If you would like a free, printable download of this protocol along with many other helpful tools and resources, please visit skinnychickweightloss.com and download it.

This will be your diet for the next three weeks. I only recommend doing up to three weeks at a time because if you do it for a very long time consecutively, your weight loss will slow down and you will very likely start retaining a lot of water. I discourage this, as it will appear you are not losing weight or in some, even that you are gaining weight. The way I like to do it and the way my clients do it is through one of these variations...

- Three weeks on rapid weight loss protocol

- One week on maintenance

- Two to three weeks on rapid loss protocol

- One week on maintenance and so on

Another variation is to do it all week and have one "cheat day" a week after the initial three weeks when starting the program. Figure out what works best for you. You will still lose weight in the maintenance phase if you do it correctly. A word on cheat days… this does not mean that you get to gorge and stuff yourself silly. Don't do it! It will drastically slow your weight loss down and you will feel awful when you do it.

You need to remember that the goal here is to relearn new habits. If you hate the way you eat all week and live only for cheat day, you are training your brain to still want junk food. The mind is powerful and the way you perceive things is powerful (we will get more into removing mental blocks to attaining the body you want in chapter 10). Be careful to work toward relearning to care about what you put in your body and see healthy food as a way to love yourself. Use the recipes in chapter 9 to figure out delicious ways to eat healthy. You will eventually prefer healthy food. This will make more sense and become more believable when you get to the maintenance portion and when you have done at least three weeks on the Skinny Chick! Rapid Fat Loss Protocol.

I know something to be true about my clients, it is one of the reasons my success rate with my clients is so high: it is easy to stick to something when you are finally getting the results you want! If you are like most of my clients, it is not that you are lazy; it is that you have done things to lose weight before but your weight loss was slow or you didn't lose weight at all. This program works, and it works quickly! That in itself helps my clients stick to it! Let's take a look at the actual Skinny Chick! Rapid Fat Loss Protocol starting on the next page.

"Every accomplishment starts with the decision to try"

Author Unknown

Skinny Chick! Rapid Fat Loss Protocol

Breakfast

Skinny Chick! Complete Protein Shake (instructions and recipes for shakes in Chapter 9)

*Or

Two-three egg omelet or eggs cooked any way, with yolks plus optional approved vegetables and a very small amount of no carbohydrate sausage

Lunch

Skinny Chick! Complete Protein Shake or two-three eggs with yolks cooked any way

Large salad with lots of leafy lettuce and up to 2 cups of small chopped approved vegetables and approved salad dressing. You may add a very small amount of almonds or sunflower seeds (3 tsp. at most) to salad for crunch if desired. A small amount of cheese (under 1 g carbohydrate per serving) may be added as well.

Dinner

Up to 8 ounces of Approved Meat

Up to 2 cups of small chopped Approved Vegetables raw or cooked

More salad if desired, but skip the nuts if you decide to have an evening salad

Snacks

Choose from…

One serving unsweetened or plain Chobani brand Greek yogurt sweetened with Stevia. Bakto flavorings may be added (find them on Amazon.com), or any flavoring as long as it does not have carbohydrates (think vanilla and other flavoring extracts). Pay attention to serving size (one serving, once daily)

Cheese stick with zero carbohydrates (once daily)

Skinny Chick! Complete Protein Shake

Half an avocado with sea salt added. You may turn it into guacamole and dip cucumber slices in it (max. ½ an avocado a day)

*If you enjoy avocados, I highly recommend you eat ½ of one a day.

½ cup of low-fat cottage cheese (not non-fat, read label), 4 g of carbohydrates or less

One to two eggs cooked any way (may be made into deviled egg, see recipes)

Any of the approved vegetables

Approved Vegetables

Alfalfa, Asparagus, Arugula, ¼ steamed Artichoke, Avocado (up to ½ day), Bell Peppers (green only), Bean Sprouts, Beet Greens, Broccoli, Brussels Sprouts (stick to 1 or less cup a day), Cauliflower, Cabbage, Celery, Chard, Chicory, Chives, Collards, Cress, Cucumbers, Edamame, Eggplant (up to 1 cup), Endive, Fennel, Green Beans, Kale, Kohlrabi, Leafy Greens, Leeks, Mushrooms, Okra, Onions (only if eaten raw and in small amounts), Hot Peppers, Pimentos, Radish, Rhubarb, Sauerkraut, Snow Peas (stick to ¼ cup or less) Spinach, Swiss Chard, Tomatoes (stick to very small serving sizes, think three to four cherry tomatoes), Turnip (stick to 1 cup or less), Watercress, Zucchini

Approved Proteins

Skinless or ground Chicken, skinless or ground Turkey (it is okay to cook chicken or turkey with the skin on. Just don't eat a lot of the skin; some is okay. Remember it has a lot of calories), Lean Beef Cuts or Ground Beef 80% fat or less, Pork Chops, any kind of Fish, Lobster, Shrimp, Oysters, Scallops, Tofu (not recommended more than twice a week), Tempeh, two to three Eggs cooked any way with yolk, Sausage (check the label, 1 g carbohydrates or less, the problem with sausage is the other ingredients added), you may splurge on a little bit of Bacon once a week (two strips or less, but eating bacon every day will add too many calories)

Approved Salad Dressing

Check the labels, as all salad dressing must be 1 g carbohydrate or under. There are some salad dressing recipes in Chapter 9.

Other Condiments and Seasonings

Apple Cider, Rice Wine or White Vinegar (no Balsamic or Red Wine, too much sugar); Dill Pickles, fresh or dried Herbs, Garlic, Ginger, Hot Sauce, Lemon/Lime Juice, Lemongrass, Mustard, Pesto (read label, 1 g carb or less), Soy Sauce, Spices, Tamari Sauce, low carb Ketchup (it has 1 g carb per serving) Vegenaise (mayonnaise replacement, find it at Whole Foods or Sprouts), 1 g or under carb Cheese may be used in moderation, dried, shakable Parmesan is okay, again in moderation. Mrs. Dash has a large line of seasonings that add a lot of flavor and are, calorie, carbohydrate, and MSG free. Stevia, Butter (in strict moderation)

*Always check labels on your condiments and spices, carbohydrates should be 0 with the exception of pickles, which must be limited to two large pickles a day, and the condiments above specifically to be kept to 1 g of carbohydrate or under. Watch your serving size.

Approved Drinks

Water, Coffee, any Unsweetened Tea, all Herbal Teas, Half and Half for Coffee or Tea, Sparkling Drinks with 0 carbohydrates and no artificial sweeteners (you can add Stevia)

If you are used to eating a lot of processed foods and the thought of eating all of these whole foods scares you, keep in mind that I include a lot of recipes in Chapter 9, as there are ways to make everything in the protocol taste good... I promise! My clients are always thrilled to have a way to make real food that tastes so good; you will feel like you are cheating. Also, keep in mind that as your body gets used to eating healthy food and you start seeing results, it gets much easier to stick to and pick healthier food options. The point of all of this is to reset your body to the point that you no longer crave junk all the time. A huge side effect of my weight loss protocol is also getting addicted to it. My clients love the results and the fact that they feel so good and full of energy! I can't tell you enough how much finally getting results will help keep you motivated!

As you will see when you look at the Skinny Chick! Rapid Fat Loss Protocol, there are three meals as well as snacks. There is a lot of food and you should not be hungry all the time once you get past the initial phase. I highly recommend taking an appetite suppressant initially, as this will help immensely until you get to the part where your body is getting a large portion of its calories from your fat cells. On Amazon.com, I sell an excellent appetite suppressant that is also an excellent thermogenic (supplement that increases fat burning) called Skinny Chick! Thermo.

As I explained, in addition to the food you are eating on the diet, you will also be getting excess calories from your fat cells, which your body will use in essentially the same way it uses carbohydrates. The great thing is that if there is excess dumped from your fat cells, it will not be re-stored in your fat cells, as excess carbohydrates are, it will be peed out. You will literally melt!

Breaking the Skinny Chick! Rapid Fat Loss Protocol Down

Let's start with breakfast: A Skinny Chick! Complete Protein Shake or a two to three egg omelet with optional approved vegetables, no carbohydrate sausage, and a very small amount of low carbohydrate cheese. I highly recommend starting the day with the shake, as it is designed to give you the right proportion of protein, carbohydrates, and fat to keep you feeling full and energized for a long time. There are recipes to vary the shakes in the recipe chapter (chapter 9), as well as the basic shake recipe.

The shake is also a very convenient way to start the day if mornings at your house are anything like they are at my house: everybody participating in the mad dash to get ready and out of the house in time for school and work. I do like the option for an omelet on the weekends though when the pace is a little slower. The omelet has a lot more calories and a lot less protein than the shake. I personally limit the omelet option to only two days or less a week. If I have eggs for breakfast, I have a shake with lunch and possibly one as a snack as well.

Now on to lunch: a large salad and a Skinny Chick! Complete Protein Shake or two to three eggs. I mean a LARGE salad here with lots of leafy greens. Stuff yourself with approved veggies. If you opt to have the Skinny Chick! Complete Protein Shake with lunch, which I recommend, you may still have an egg on your salad if you like that. As you know from what I have explained, you are dumping toxins out of your fat cells along with the fat. Your daily salad will act as a broom sweeping through your intestines to get the toxins out of your body thus avoiding a build-up of toxins that will slow down or even halt your weight loss until your body can get rid of them.

Avoid iceberg lettuce, or at least don't eat it with any regularity. It has very little nutrient content and is actually known to cause constipation, as opposed to help clean out your intestines, like leafy lettuces do. You will very likely get tired of salads. Taking a break from them and replacing them with just the approved veggies is fine from time to time. Just ensure that you get in a salad most days. You may also have your salad for dinner instead of lunch if you prefer (swapping lunch and dinner is fine). Add a salad dressing that makes your salad taste good. The only thing you need to worry about with salad dressing is making sure it has 1 g of carbohydrate or under, stick to the serving size, and make sure it does not contain corn syrup. The reason I say no corn syrup is that it has many negative effects on the body, most notably a negative effect on your pancreas. I question how a salad dressing can remain under 1 carbohydrate if it has corn syrup in it but somehow I have found salad dressings that claim to have under a gram of carbohydrate yet still contain the nasty stuff.

Get in the habit of reading labels. I will get much more into the whys of not eating all of the extra artificial preservatives, colors, and additives so prevalent in the food at the grocery store in the maintenance section of this book, so read on. Basically, the less added "junk" it has in it, the better. If the dressing you pick up has a list a mile long of ingredients you can't pronounce on it, put it back… we are not meant to eat things like that with regularity. One good line of dressings that has a lot of 1 g of carbohydrate or under choices is called Marie's, and you can get it in most grocery stores by the refrigerated salad dressings. They are very good and have no artificial preservatives and natural ingredients.

Another good brand I have discovered in the refrigerated section is Marzetti Simply Dressed. Search around; I am sure you will find a lot of options in these parameters! I have the most luck finding dressings I like to consume in the refrigerated dressings section. There are also good ones in the condiment section of the grocery store.

Many salad dressings do contain soybean oil and canola oil, which I do not love but unless you are allergic to soy, the amount you will get from 2 tablespoons of salad dressing is not going to hurt you and a delicious salad dressing makes a delicious salad, so splurge in this area!

I recommend adding some avocado to your salad daily if you like avocados. As I mention throughout the book, I am a big fan and consider them a super food. They also add a delicious creamy texture to whatever you are eating. One thing I also do is add a little bit of the parmesan chips (found in chapter 9) crumbled up on top of my salad. It adds a crunchy texture, which I love on a salad, as well as great flavor and zero carbohydrates. Get into a salad a day as often as you can do it habit. It's a habit your body will thank you for! Don't eat boring, plain salads with nothing on them… get creative, make your salads delicious and change them up daily. When people see my salads, they say 'Yum!' Your salad does not have to be and should not be boring!

I tend to make dinner the heaviest meal of my day. In the evening, I wind down and get ready to turn in for the night as most people do. This is also when most people are the most hungry. It makes sense for me to prepare the biggest and heaviest meal of the day after work and before I relax. If this is not true for you, find what works for you. You may rearrange the meals to suit what works best for you without hurting your results. Try to eat your last meal before 7:00 pm, but if you can't do that then don't fret too much. Eating before 7:00 pm will normally ensure that your digestion of a big meal will not impede sleep. Meat can be consumed every night for dinner if you want. This makes me personally feel like I get a big, substantial meal when I like to eat my big, substantial meal. You do not however, need to consume meat at all. The meat may be replaced with a Skinny Chick! Complete Protein Shake or two to three eggs. Just ensure you get a minimum of one Skinny Chick! Complete Protein Shake in a day.

Finally snacks… snacking is okay throughout the entire Skinny Chick! Rapid Fat Loss Protocol if needed. However, consider this: in between meals is when your body will be burning the largest amount of fat, as your body will have no other source for energy when there is no other option. In other words, you do have to eat real food to fuel your body; your body will not just live on ketones alone. Right after you eat a meal, your body will have the calories it needs to use up before it can go back to burning fat as energy. A longer amount of time without snacks in between breakfast, lunch and dinner will mean a higher amount of fat being turned into energy or fat melting off of you. That being said, some people have a higher metabolism or need the extra calories of the snacks between each meal. That is fine; just don't eat the snacks if you don't "need" them. I personally never need one in between breakfast and lunch and sometimes but not always need one between lunch and dinner, depending on how active I have been that day while on protocol. It is wise to always have a snack handy in case you do need one; however, you do not want to get to the point where you are so hungry you are tempted to cheat. Figure out what works best for you.

Protein

Let's discuss protein, as it is a very important component of being on a fat loss diet. Remember at the beginning I told you that if you do this perfectly, you will lose very little of your muscle mass, which is a large factor in your metabolic rate. The goal of this diet is to retain as much muscle mass as possible and lose primarily fat. To do that, you need to eat adequate protein that the body absorbs well. The reason I do not have meat listed at every meal is that meat is not a readily absorbed protein. Depending on the person and how good their digestion is, the body will absorb about 50–68% or less of the protein in meat. The rest of it will be spilled over into your kidneys to be excreted.

The big issue with this is that your kidneys are already working at an accelerated rate processing and getting rid of all the toxins pouring out of your fat cells. The protein that goes through your kidneys is acidic; if this gets backed up, you will get excess acidity in your body and your body will shut down dumping fat until it gets itself to a proper pH level again. This is why I recommend consuming eggs and my low carbohydrate, high protein Skinny Chick! Complete Protein Shake. The protein in eggs is almost 100% absorbed; however, they have about 6 g of protein per egg, not a large enough amount.

I am not typically a proponent of "meal replacement" options, as I feel they are usually packed with sugar and artificial preservatives, which you will understand by now goes against your goals while you are trying to lose weight and heal your body. That is why my shake is made with very high quality whey protein. My low carbohydrate (2 g per serving), high protein (26 g per serving), under 1 g sugar (sweetened with Stevia) Skinny Chick! Super Whey Protein Mix can be purchased on Amazon.com. I tried so many protein mixes in my search for creating a high protein, low carbohydrate protein shake for my program that I could not possibly count them all. The one made for my program is simply the best! It is creamy, mixes well (no nasty clumps in your shake), it is smooth (not grainy), and is an incredible value compared to other brands that can sell at twice the price of my mix. It also comes in three delicious flavors: vanilla, strawberry, and chocolate. More information about my Skinny Chick! Super Whey Protein Mix in chapter 8.

More on Whey Protein

Why Whey Protein when there are so many different kinds of protein supplements out there? I'm often asked: why did I choose Whey? For starters, you need a protein that is very absorbable; almost all of the protein in whey protein isolate is absorbed by the body. Whey protein is also the king of muscle building proteins. Studies have shown that whey protein increases muscle protein synthesis (muscle building) by a whopping 70%! Other proteins tested yielded a measly 30% increase or under. Ladies, don't be afraid to build muscle; this will not cause you to turn into a body builder. Remember that muscle is highly metabolically active and needs calories even when you are holding still. The more muscle you have, the more fat you burn at all times! I also find whey protein to have a high safety profile. For example: I believe soy protein to be disruptive to our hormones, in particular estrogen. To my knowledge, there is simply nothing like that with whey protein. The whey protein used specifically for this program (Skinny Chick! Super Whey Protein Mix) is 100% whey protein isolate, meaning that it is lactose free. It is also guaranteed to be free from MSG and other exitototixins. In my opinion, whey is also the smoothest and best tasting protein supplement on the market. One more big reason I chose whey is that it boosts glutathione levels. Glutathione is the most important antioxidant our body possesses. It has been dubbed "the master antioxidant" because it keeps all the other antioxidants in your body working properly by basically regenerating them. Glutathione is found in every cell in your body.

Unfortunately, with the poor diets so many have, low glutathione levels have become all too common. This leaves your cells more susceptible to damage by free radicals. There are many, many glutathione supplements on the market; however, glutathione has been proven to be poorly absorbed through the digestive system. This basically means that these supplements are a huge waste of money. The best way to boost your glutathione levels is to give your body the precursors or ingredients it needs to create its own glutathione. Boosting your glutathione levels boosts every other antioxidant in your body, which is especially important while you are detoxing (such as when you are on the Skinny

Chick! Rapid Fat Loss Protocol). The toxins released while you are detoxing can behave as free radicals, thus causing cell damage. Whey protein is the absolute best when it comes to boosting glutathione levels. It contains all the precursors necessary for the body to make glutathione, as well as another special cysteine residue called glutamylcysteine, which is instrumental in converting these precursors into glutathione. It is important to use 100% whey protein isolate that is processed in a way that creates a very pure protein without damaging the precursors rendering them useless, such as my Skinny Chick! Super Whey Protein Mix, which can be found on Amazon.com. The full scope of the ways that high glutathione levels and whey protein will enhance your health and weight loss are beyond the scope of this book. I highly encourage you to research it further and see for yourself!

Adequate amounts of the correct protein is essential for the Skinny Chick! Rapid Fat Loss Protocol. You must have at least one Skinny Chick! Complete Protein Shake a day (found in recipes in chapter 9) to have success in this program. The clients who get the best results have two to three Skinny Chick! Complete Protein Shakes a day. The reason the clients who have multiple shakes a day get better results is in part, as I have already mentioned, that muscle is a fat burner in of itself. It is not biologically inactive like fat is; it does not just hang out and take up space. The more muscle you have, the more you burn fat even when you are doing absolutely nothing. As you already know if you read the section on whey protein above, good whey protein is a superb muscle building protein. This means that as your body is burning fat as its main energy source while you are in ketosis, if you are consuming whey protein and building muscle, your new muscle mass will also be using fat from your fat cells for the energy it needs. More muscle equals faster fat burning.

The other reason it is essential is that you need to protect your muscle mass. Remember earlier in the book, I explained that our body likes to use food for energy in this order: carbohydrates, protein, and then fat. Well now that your body is burning fat and using it as it would normally use carbohydrates, you are basically bypassing your body's need to use carbohydrates as its primary energy source while melting your fat stores. However, in the body, it is a long, drawn out biological process to turn fat into an end product that mimics a carbohydrate (ketones). If your body starts to need more energy because it can't make this breakdown happen quickly enough, what do you think your body will go for? It will go for your muscle mass, as you are not eating a lot of carbohydrates, your body's preferred source of easy energy (the brain and kidneys will use what you are eating).

Consuming adequate muscle building protein, such as Skinny Chick! Super Whey Protein Mix, will ensure your body has plenty of protein as its back up source of energy and will build muscle, thus boosting calorie and fat burning. Do not neglect your protein shakes, your results will not be the same without them!

Fat

Now, let's talk about fat. I was delighted to see a segment on *The Today Show* at the end of 2014 daring to ask the question: is fat really bad for you? Does it really cause heart disease? Mark my words; you will start seeing a lot more stories like this in mainstream media! Fat is arguably the most misunderstood nutrient there is. The low fat diet craze has caused much more harm than good, as it has replaced fats with carbohydrates (specifically sugar and over-refined carbohydrates, such as white bread), as well as caused other health issues that I will touch on in a moment. This myth has all but been completely debunked with all of the recent studies, yet I still see nutritionists and doctors on TV and in articles pushing a low fat and specifically low-saturated fat, often high-carbohydrate diet.

I recently overheard people in an elevator discussing how they wished avocados were good for you because they would eat them all the time but they are too high in fat! I eat on average, half of if not a whole avocado almost every day because not only are they healthy, they are a super food! So what is going on here? How did this myth get so out of control? It all started with a flawed study done by Dr. Keys in 1958. The study compared six countries and their prevalence for heart disease compared with their fat consumption statistics. From this study, Dr. Keys concluded that there was a direct correlation between the six countries' fat consumption statistics and heart disease.

Upon further investigation of this study (years later), it was found that there were actually statistics for twenty-two countries and when those statistics were added into the analysis, the fat-to-heart disease correlation disappeared. Unfortunately, this is a perfect example of a fatal flaw in so many studies we use to prove health facts and follow blindly. It is an all too often harmful trend that a study "proves" an outcome and the combination of the study and powerful marketing by food and pharmaceutical companies turns it into truth. It appeared when Dr. Keys work was looked into later; he truly believed that his theory was correct. So much so that he may have skewed the study so the outcome would prove his theory correct by leaving out the statistics of the countries that disproved his theory. Unfortunately, no matter how much proof there is to the contrary, myths that gain popularity and are adopted as the absolute truth by the public take a long time to undo.

Take cigarettes as an example. Everybody knows they are bad for you and that they cause cancer but did you know that sixty years after that was proven, marketing companies and some doctors were still touting them as healthy? A large advertisement campaign by the tobacco companies depicted their brands as ones that doctors recommend.

It may take time to undo the notion that fat and in particular, the cholesterol in some fat is the most evil thing in nutrition… but it will happen. There are simply too many reliable studies being done for it not to take hold eventually. Interestingly enough, one thing that came out of this belief is a huge push for using certain vegetable oils that contain trans-fat, such as the ones found in margarine and vegetable shortening. It has been discovered now that trans-fats are the true health stealing, heart-disease-causing bad fat culprits as they both raise LDL (bad cholesterol) and lower HDL (good cholesterol that helps keep bad cholesterol in control). Despite this, I still see commercials advertising the healthy alternative to butter. Guess what, these for the most part are not healthy alternatives. As a matter of fact, butter in moderation is just fine, even healthy. Organic is better and we will get to why in chapter 5.

Scientists have discovered two types of saturated fat: one particle is small and dense (the kind linked to heart disease), and one is large and fluffy (this kind appears to do no harm). This subject is simply too complicated to cover in this book. Science is also constantly changing and evolving, as people are able to look at old studies that were turned into "truth" more subjectively and find issues that were never seen before as well as conduct more accurate studies.

I want you to take this from it though: do not be afraid of fat. Fat is not your enemy. Refined carbohydrates are and you need to train your body to not want them anymore to achieve your health and weight loss goals. Your body will thank you with better health, more energy, and weight loss!

Fat will help you lose weight… yes help you. It will keep you satisfied; it will make things taste good; it will keep you full; and it will help you not crave sugar and refined carbohydrates. In fact, while people are on my program, if I get the complaint that they are still very hungry at night and particularly craving sugar at night, I will examine their food journal. Upon examination of their food journal, it is almost always one of three things: not enough water, not enough protein, or not enough fat. The latter is almost always the culprit. Helping them find ways to incorporate more fat almost always reverses it. The exception is when there is a habit that has been created by eating sweets every night. More on how to get past this later in the book.

Incorporate good fats into your diet: add oil or even a little bit of butter (a lot of butter will still equal a lot of calories) to your vegetables to make them taste good. Eat spoonfuls of coconut oil if you are craving sugar and watch your sugar craving disappear. Include avocados in your diet as often as possible. Make dipping sauces for your meat with ingredients that contain good fat. Seek out the new research on fat, including saturated fat and educate yourself. One thing my clients say they are most happy about taking away from this program is that they no longer fear fat. Opt for 35–40% of your diet being healthy fat or more. Examples of healthy fat are listed below.

Some Examples of Fats to Include in Your Diet

- Coconut Oil
- Organic Fatty Meat
- Olive Oil
- Organic Egg Yolks
- Organic Butter in moderation

- Palm Oil

- Nuts

- Nut Oils

- Avocados

- Grapeseed Oil

- Animal Based Omega 3 Supplement (plant based Omega 3 supplements are not absorbed as well)

Some Examples of Fats to Avoid in Your Diet

- Margarine

- Canola Oil (too much Omega 6, which blocks Omega 3 fatty acids)

- Crisco

- Any Kind of Vegetable Shortening

- Partially Hydrogenated Oil

- Deep Fried Foods

- Non-Organic Fatty Meat (Explained in the case for Organic chapter, chapter 5)

Now that we have covered fat a little bit, let's talk about cheese. I find people are surprised that I include some cheese in my diet. Is cheese a health food in my opinion? Maybe some very natural and quality cheeses are in moderation but overall no, I do not think cheese can be considered a health food. So why do I include it on the program?! You already know that I do not think fat is the dietary issue it has been made out to be, so I do not see the fat in cheese as an issue. I see cheese as a very low or no carbohydrate way to add both fat, which will keep you full and satisfied longer, as well as the fact that it makes things taste better!

When you start making some of the meals found in the recipes in Chapter 9 of this book, you will discover that some of them are so good, it feels like you are cheating on your diet but they are perfectly within protocol! That sure makes it much easier to stick to the program and achieve your weight loss goals right?! Don't be afraid to add in some cheese. However, cheese is high in calories so don't over-do it.

While I do not think weight loss is as simple as calories in versus calories out, keeping your calories reasonably low while in the rapid fat loss portion of your diet will enhance your results. If you like Parmesan cheese, that is a good choice to add flavor, as it is a very strong flavored cheese and does not take much to add flavor. If you are lactose intolerant, you may still be able to enjoy a little bit of cheese. An easy way to tell if you will able to tolerate a cheese is to look at the nutrition label. Cheese that has zero carbohydrates will also be very low or devoid of lactose (and will be the best for protocol anyway). Many people who otherwise cannot handle dairy can often handle small amounts of some cheeses. Aged cheeses like Cheddar, Swiss, and Parmesan, all tend to be inherently low in lactose. You can get a supplement at any health food store called lactase. Lactase is the enzyme you need to break down lactose. Many people who are intolerant of dairy foods find that if they take lactase with a small amount of low lactose dairy food, such as cheese, they no longer have the negative side effects that lactose intolerance can cause.

Required Supplements

Some supplements are absolutely required to be on this program:

- Whey Protein: we covered this before, my Skinny Chick! Super Whey Protein Supplement is the best for this program and can be purchased at my online store at Amazon.com.

- Potassium: I will cover the whys of this supplement as we go. It is not optional while on program and it is not an expensive supplement. I chose Now brand Potassium Citrate 99 mg for my program which can be purchased on Amazon.com and many health food stores and will give you the exact right amount and type of potassium for this program.

- Real Sea Salt: this will also be covered more in the supplements section. I get mine at Sprouts but it can be found on Amazon.com as well. It is called Real Salt and it is inexpensive and very high in quality.

- Calcium and Magnesium Supplements: this will also be covered in greater length later on. Skinny Chick! Calcium Magnesium can be purchased on Amazon.com and is the perfect one for this program.

There are other supplements that I highly recommend. Much more information on the required supplements and the recommended ones in chapter 8.

Alcohol and Other Beverages That Are Not Okay

I will be honest with you, most of my clients do not like this part but drinking alcohol of any kind does not belong in a weight loss and body-healing program. Don't get me wrong, I love my vino but I do not think it is appropriate for every night consumption and I have seen so many people do everything right on my protocol but they can't stick to this one thing, and their results are never as good as the people who follow this rule. Aside from the fact that even if your drink of choice has zero carbohydrates, it still has an effect on your pancreas, your liver and your weight loss.

Alcohol tends to make most people crave simple carbohydrates. Most of all, it adds to the acidity of your body. Your body has to keep itself at a proper pH. As I have said before, if you throw your body into an acidic state, it will halt dumping fat out of your cells and not start again until it has balanced out your pH.

I also want you to avoid soda, even diet soda. While a diet soda here and there will not destroy your fat loss, it will again slow it down. Part of this goes back to the pH issue, soda makes your body very acidic and your body will need to mitigate that before it can move back into fat burning mode.

Another issue that needs to be addressed with any kind of a weight loss program: artificial sweeteners. Avoid them as much as possible, as they will lead to sugar cravings among other things. I get more into artificial sweeteners in chapter 4. You may use Stevia to sweeten things. More on where to get the best Stevia in Chapter 8.

Why No Dessert and Why No Fruit?

I get this question so often. The answer is simple but I will elaborate: too much sugar! As far as dessert goes, I understand that some programs include a dessert made up entirely of artificial chemicals and artificial sweeteners so that you don't have to miss your dessert. After you read this book in its entirety, you will understand why that is not a good thing but for now, let's just examine this point: do you want to stay in the habit of eating dessert every night?

This is about more than weight loss; this is about changing your body chemistry and habits so you can be free of these sorts of cravings for good. Can you imagine not being interested in having a dessert at night? Can you imagine not craving sugar anymore? You won't get there if you keep supporting that habit so start now to break free from it.

I go over some useful tips on how to overcome cravings until you get your body to the point where you don't want these things anymore and yes, it will take some will power on your part before you can get there. Isn't that worth it though? I don't refrain from dessert at all times personally but it takes very little to satisfy me if I do reach for something sweet. Best of all, I do not even think about or want anything sugary for the most part and I used to eat up to a bag of family sized M&Ms a day! In fact, I used to be unbelievably addicted to sugar. So this is not coming from a person who has never had a serious affinity for the stuff… this is coming from a person who has found a way to no longer want the stuff. Sugar is a drug in food form. If you are craving it, you have set your body up to crave it by throwing off your body chemistry. This can and will be reversed! Follow my tips for getting past these cravings in the beginning and get yourself to the point where you no longer need it. It is one of the best things I have ever done for my health.

As far as fruit goes, fruit is wonderful. I love fruit. I keep it around the house for all of us to snack on. However, it is called nature's candy for a reason. That reason is that it is chock full of sugar. Yes, it has many health benefits, vitamins, minerals, and phytonutrients; that simply can't be denied. While you are losing weight however, it will halt your efforts in their tracks. Keep in mind that maintaining your healthy goal weight is dramatically easier than losing weight. In other words, fruit is not out forever, just for now.

One way that I add a fruity flavor to my life when I am in protocol mode is to flavor my plain Chobani Greek yogurt with it. There is a line of natural flavorings called Bakto Flavors that you can get on Amazon.com. They have a long list of flavors. In my office, I currently carry Vanilla, Caramel, Chocolate, Orange, Mango, Coconut, Strawberry, and Pumpkin Spice. This nowhere approaches their entire line. They are tasty and they can be added to your shake or plain Greek yogurt with no ill effect on your results. You can also find flavorings in many grocery stores… just be careful and read your labels. If the alcohol they use in many flavorings as a preservative is a concern to you, heat your flavoring up, as this will make the alcohol dissolve out of the flavoring. There is not enough alcohol content to hinder your results unless you use it in serious excess.

Water

The importance of consuming enough water, especially while on protocol cannot be overstated! Water, water and more water... water is your new best friend! Take your weight in pounds and divide it by two, you should be drinking a minimum of this number in ounces a day. While trying to lose weight; however, you should consume much more, about 8–10 ounces or more per every 10 pounds you want to lose. The fat will not leave your cells and flush out through your lymphatic and eliminatory system if there is not enough water to move it out. If you don't drink enough water, you will not lose weight; it is as simple as that!

Remember that you will also be flushing toxins out of your fat cells, so water will also help flush all of these toxins out of your body. Lemon or lime juice can be added to your water while on protocol and is recommended, as it is very alkalizing. You may also put water in a pitcher with sliced cucumbers overnight to make cucumber water, which is very refreshing. There is a product called Electro Mix by Emergen-C. It is a drink mix that comes in packets that turns your water into a sports drink with no sugar and a refreshing lemon-lime flavor. It is a great way to flavor water while on protocol if you get tired of plain water and it contains potassium and magnesium along with other minerals.

You can also drink as much herbal tea as you wish while on protocol and there are a lot of wonderful flavors to choose from. I enjoy iced herbal teas in the summer. If you are a coffee or caffeinated tea drinker, caffeinated drinks do not count toward your overall fluid consumption as they act as a diuretic. Get in the habit of drinking water all the time… your entire body will thank you for it!

Chapter 3
What to Expect While Getting Started

Your body will be undergoing a radical and quick shift, especially if you have been eating a lot of highly processed junk food all your life. This can cause temporary side effects, which we will go over in detail, as well as how to combat the side effects. Some people experience every side effect horribly and some don't experience any side effects. Most experience some of them just mildly. All side effects are temporary and treatable. If something very strange happens to you that seems scary or dangerous, stop the diet and consult with your doctor. Do remember though that this is just food. Although food can be a powerful tool for healing, healthy food is not something that will harm you.

If you have kidney issues, you should not do the Skinny Chick! Rapid Fat Loss portion of the diet. If you are on any medication, your doctor should monitor you. Medications in particular are those for high blood pressure and type 2 diabetes, as well as for hypothyroidism. Your doctor will need to monitor you, as your dosage will likely need to be lowered as you progress on this program if you are on blood pressure or type 2 diabetes medication. Failing to do so can cause serious health issues and make you feel terrible, so make sure you pay attention to this. If you have hypothyroidism that is not controlled properly, you can have issues on this program, as it "can" slow your thyroid down further. People with hypothyroidism may be wise to do a week on Skinny Chick! Rapid Fat Loss Protocol and a week off while having your levels monitored by your doctor and or watching out for low thyroid symptoms.

Pregnant women should never do this program under any circumstances. Nursing women will not produce enough milk if they do this program while still nursing but may do the maintenance portion until they are finished nursing. If you have any health condition whatsoever and are unsure as to whether you should be on a diet that makes you lose weight this quickly, consult your doctor! Do not take any chances with doing this incorrectly and hurting yourself. You always have the option to do a modified version of this protocol where you do not actually go into ketosis. This will not yield results as quickly but if you can't do it safely, do not do it.

I want this to be a wonderful journey to empowerment for you. I want you to learn that you hold the key to your health and well-being. For the most part, you will feel amazing on the Complete Rapid Weight Loss Protocol. The first three days to week however, can be uncomfortable for some, especially if you have had a diet full of junk before you start this. Most people have their worst day on day three to four due to the fact that you will likely have reached the end of your glycogen stores (the carbohydrates stored in your muscles and liver that your body must burn through before it will start using the fat in your fat cells for energy) and will be converting to ketosis (using fat from your fat cells as energy instead of carbohydrates) at this time. I recommend extra rest on day three to four if you can do that and know that when you get into ketosis, you will know because you will feel much better, even amazing! You will start to have more energy and less hunger. Here is a list of the things that you may experience while you are getting started.

Herxheimer's Reaction

I will start with an explanation that will cover some of the reason you may experience most of the symptoms below. Herxheimer's Reaction, also known as a healing response, is your body's response to either rapid healing or a rapid killing off of pathogens. Most people have an overgrowth of bad pathogens or parasites in their body to some degree. If you have been eating anything that converts quickly to glucose in your body, you have been feeding the little "bad" critters in your gut. Now, by cutting fast glucose food out of your diet, you have suddenly cut off their food supply, which will make them start dying off rapidly. These pathogens, like all living creatures, do not want to die. To try to stop you from killing them, they start letting off chemicals that can cause many of the symptoms below.

Our bodies actually have more bacteria than cells. We should have a good bacteria to bad bacteria ratio in our gut of approximately 80–85% good to 15–20% bad. Most people have a much different ratio with the bad bacteria being dominant... this is called dysbiosis. This can cause many health issues, including an inability to lose weight, as well as excess gas and bloating. All the implications of not having a correct ratio of good to bad bacteria are beyond the scope of this text. You are getting the excess bad guys down to a normal level while on my protocol and this is a very good thing. In Chapter 8, I will recommend a good probiotic to help cultivate more good bacteria in your gut so that you may work toward a healthier bacteria ratio.

Headaches

This is a classic Herxheimer's Reaction symptom but while on protocol, it can mean other things as well. When you seriously restrict fast burning glucose foods, your body will rapidly stop producing too much insulin. This can and will cause your kidneys to dump the excess insulin it has been storing, bringing sodium and potassium along with magnesium with it. This sudden drop of sodium and potassium in your body can lead to low blood pressure and dizziness. Be absolutely sure to get enough salt in the first few days. In fact, it may be prudent to have extra salt and potassium on days two to five to be sure you are getting enough sodium and potassium. See instructions on how to do this in Chapter 8. If you have a headache that is caused by this, it should be relieved in fifteen to twenty minutes by a salt shot (explanation of salt shots in Chapter 8) and a big glass of water with potassium.

It is also very important that you take your potassium supplements throughout the entire protocol and at the elevated levels outlined in Chapter 8 while you are starting the Skinny Chick! Rapid Fat Loss Protocol. If you are on medication for high blood pressure, you will need to monitor your blood pressure carefully, as the combination of this protocol and medication to lower your blood pressure may make your blood pressure too low. Some find that they need to lower their dose of medication or discontinue it all together (consult with your doctor). If you have a stubborn headache that just will not go away, you may take a painkiller to get through it or sniff peppermint essential oil and put it on your temples diluted with olive or coconut oil. For most people who experience this side effect, it is manageable and goes away within the first three days to one week.

Fatigue

Another classic Herxheimer's Reaction symptom; this can also be caused by low blood pressure covered under headaches or due to low blood sugar. It is a shock to your body to all of a sudden take away its easy source of energy (fast burning glucose foods), and it takes a couple of days for your body to get to the point where it is using the ketonic bodies (your melting fat) as its primary source of energy. Once it does, you will feel amazing, so hang in there. Get extra rest if you can, consume extra caffeine if you need to.

Hunger

Now, I know you are saying, 'Wait, you said I would not be hungry!' That is true; however, it again takes a few days for your body to convert to using your fat for fuel. Until then, you may experience hunger. I sell an excellent supplement that works both as an appetite suppressant and a thermogenic called Skinny Chick! Thermo on Amazon.com. You need to make sure you eat all of your meals and snacks at reasonable times and stay ahead of your hunger. If you are hungry, eat something, just make sure it is within protocol. If you need extra protocol food to get through the initial phase, that is fine. Do not go hungry.

Nausea

Yet again, classic Herxheimer's Reaction; this is also caused by the shock your body can experience from such a drastic change in your diet. This diet changes your metabolism and the way your body handles food. The transition can take a few days, so hang in there. Ginger tea is excellent for getting rid of nausea and tastes delicious too. You can add Stevia to it if you need it sweetened, but do not use honey.

Muscle Cramps

This is again due to the fact that your body will start dumping excess insulin along with sodium and potassium. Make sure you are taking your potassium and salt shots correctly and you may double your potassium if needed temporarily, as outlined in Chapter 8. Taking a mega dose of your potassium should alleviate symptoms in thirty to forty-five minutes. All of your large muscle contractions, including your heart beating, require sodium and potassium so be vigilant in taking your salt and potassium, especially in the first week.

Diarrhea or Constipation

Both symptoms are possibly the most classic Herxheimer's Reaction symptoms. If you are prone to constipation, you will need to be preemptive because this will most likely cause constipation if you are already prone to it. Make sure you are drinking a ton of water, and you can buy an herbal tea or supplement called Smooth Move from the health food store and most grocery stores. You can also buy Smooth Move in capsule form on Amazon.com. If you take any other supplements for constipation, read the label and watch out for carbohydrates. You must keep your bowels moving; if you do not, your weight loss will slow way down or stop completely. Toxins and wastes that you have been exposed to over the years that your body could not get rid of are stored in your fat cells as we covered previously. If your body has no way to get rid of these toxins, it will not release them or the fat surrounding them in your fat cells.

Diarrhea is simply your body throwing dead pathogens and wastes out of your body, as quickly as it can. I do not recommend slowing it down unless it is excessive, as this can cause your body to redistribute wastes. Diarrhea is much less common on this protocol and will pass.

Bad Breath

Also a Herxheimer's Reaction symptom and it can be caused by the ketonic bodies that can cause a metallic taste in your mouth initially. Only one to two pieces of sugar-free gum can be consumed per day (some people will be kicked out of ketosis by even sugar-free gum). I personally use a breath spray that can be purchased at the health food store called Herbal Breath Tonic and it can be used as often as needed. Peppermint tea is another way to have fresh breath, get some extra fluid in, and it tastes great. Peppermint oil is one more good option, and a small drop of it is strong and will freshen your breath right up!

Bloating

Toward the end of the initial three weeks or even after the first week, some dieters start to notice some water retention. Theories abound as to why this happens to some in ketosis. I know that it is annoying, as it makes it very difficult to see your results. Be certain you are drinking plenty of water. If your body does not feel it has enough water, it will retain water. You may also want to consider taking a very mild diuretic to help shed the excess water weight to help keep you motivated (and just to relieve the discomfort). My very mild and very safe, yet effective diuretic formula with all of the best natural diuretic ingredients called Skinny Chick! Bloat Eraser is available in my Amazon.com store.

Additional Tips

- Plan ahead: if you are hungry and you still need to go to the store, take the food home and prepare it; what do you think the chances you will stick to the protocol will be? This sort of diet takes more preparation but once you have done it for a week, you will be addicted to how it makes you feel to eat this way. On top of that, your fat will start to melt off! Pack your lunch the night before and take it to work with you. The shakes can also be made the night before. Chop massive amounts of vegetables for the week for your salad on Sunday night or whenever you have time and put them in Tupperware. Consider investing in a food processor to make chopping go faster. Stay on top of your hunger, and try not to wait until you are starving to figure out what you are going to eat.

- Stay ahead of your hunger: this ties in with planning ahead. If you wait until you are starving, it will take some serious will power not to break protocol

- Don't go to the store hungry... ever! It will make your life so difficult. Items that did not even sound good before will sound awesome if you are hungry.

- Don't keep unhealthy food in your house. The excuse I get the most...I have it in there for my kids or significant other. All I can say to that is do you really want your kids or your significant other eating that stuff either?

- Keep healthy, protocol friendly snacks in your house and with you, ready to eat. If they are there and you are hungry, you will be more likely to pick them than if you have to go get them at the store.

- If you have a craving, really ask yourself: am I really hungry or am I bored, upset, angry, or just keeping a nasty habit going? Drink a big glass of water or tea, go for a walk, do something else, and it will go away. I know that sounds too simple to work but doing something else and getting your mind off of it will most likely make you forget about it. Remember, the longer you maintain your healthy habits, the less your body will have these cravings. It is worth it to get to a point where these cravings are a thing of the past, believe me!

- Don't listen to other people if they tell you what you are doing is crazy. It is always a good thing to take care of yourself, love yourself, and adopt healthy habits. It is not vain or selfish to want to look and feel good in your own skin. Don't let people talk you out of your newfound healthy lifestyle. Only you have to live in your body. Please take the time to do the exercises in Chapter 10 of this book to help get past your mental blocks, including other people, to losing weight.

- Write everything you eat down in your food journal which you can download for free at skinnychickweightloss.com that way you can go back through it if you are unsure if you are doing it correctly or have me go through it if you are participating in one of my programs. This will also help you remember if you have had certain things day to day.

- Don't work-out strenuously while on Skinny Chick! Rapid Fat Loss Protocol. There will be no glycogen in your muscles, which will cause two things to happen: you will both not feel good and it will burn muscle. Walking, doing light free weight lifting, squats, yoga, or other light workouts are okay but anything more should be saved for when you are in maintenance. I am a HUGE advocate of exercise and I absolutely endorse moving your body strenuously when you are done with the Skinny Chick! Rapid Fat Loss Protocol to help you maintain your new, slimmer figure. Working out strenuously while in the rapid fat loss phases will slow your weight loss down... I have seen it over and over again. Please read more about exercise while on and off the rapid fat loss protocol in Chapter 7.

- Eat everything on this protocol and do not skip meals. If you don't eat enough calories, your body will think you are starving and slow your metabolism way down. You are also much more likely to be able to stick to healthy food if you are not starving. Starving yourself is never ever a healthy or appropriate way to lose weight. Our bodies need fuel; we just need the correct fuel. If you are hungry, by all means eat something; just eat something that is on protocol.

- Start cutting back on caffeine. While you are in ketosis is a great time to do it because you will have an increase in energy after you get past the initial stages. Some caffeine is okay but it needs to be consumed in moderation. I personally love my daily cup of joe but I limit it to one to two cups and try not to consume any more than that.

- You can absolutely sweeten things with Stevia but try to stick to five servings or less a day... any more than that and you can end up going over the limit possibly kicking yourself out of ketosis.

- Remember, this part is temporary. When you get to your goal weight, you can eat whatever you want in moderation. Our bodies do not want to lose weight due to the fact that we are still hard-wired for survival, it is unnatural! Maintaining your weight is infinitely easier than losing weight!

- Never ever shake hot liquids in your blender bottle (you will need one to make the Skinny Chick! Complete Protein Shake). If you do, when you open the spout, it will go everywhere, burning you and making a mess.

- If you are taking contraceptives, this diet can cause them not to work or not work as well temporarily. This is hypothetical but it can happen so a backup method is advised!

- Take care of yourself... get extra rest if you need it. Remember, this is a huge metabolic shift for your body; until your body is used to it, it may gripe a little bit. The path to wellness can sometimes cause some discomfort initially. Keep your eye on the prize and look forward to how amazing you are going to look and feel after these initial few days.

- Do not cheat! If you cheat while you are on protocol weeks, you will not only <u>not get</u> the results you want, you will lower your metabolism and when you go back to your old ways, you will pack the pounds back on plus some! This is temporary, and if you follow it perfectly, you will get fast results. What you get out of this program and how good your results are is up to you. If you cheat, you are only cheating yourself.

- There is a product called Miracle Noodles that you may eat while on protocol that may be purchased on iherb.com or Amazon.com. They smell funny when you open them but once you rinse them and cook them they taste like whatever you put on them. Check recipes (chapter 9) for some ideas for Miracle Noodles recipes.

- If in a rush, pick up a rotisserie chicken and some veggies for an easy meal. You can also go out to eat, but just eat meat and veggies. Tokyo Joes is a great place to get simply prepared meats and vegetables that will keep you on protocol. Prepare your own food as often as possible so that you know what you are eating!

- You can switch lunch and dinner when needed (when going out to lunch, etc.)

- Things called Ketostix can be found at Walgreens, Rite Aide, or on Amazon.com to monitor when you go into ketosis. Be warned though, after a few weeks, your body will use the ketonic bodies more efficiently and you may no longer register on the sticks. This does not mean you are not in ketosis anymore, just the opposite. Some people never register on the Ketostix yet they are still in ketosis.

Chapter 4
Maintaining Your Weight Loss

When coming off of the protocol, do not come off with a big carbohydrate rich meal and or alcohol. Depending on how long you have been on protocol, this can make you feel very sick! I have had clients in the past not heed this warning and they ended up vomiting or just feeling really crappy for a couple days. Your pancreas has been on idle while you have been on this protocol, so introducing fast burning glucose foods will make your pancreas "wake up" suddenly, which can be unpleasant if you give it too much to process. Your body will also be more sensitive to alcohol in its new detoxified state. When coming off of the Skinny Chick! Rapid Fat Loss Protocol, especially if you do three full weeks of it; have two of the following choices a couple mornings in a row for breakfast then eat according to the protocol the rest of the day without as much worry about getting too many carbohydrates…

- A large piece of fruit

- One piece of whole grain toast with butter or peanut butter

- Low sugar yogurt

- Add a Skinny Chick! Complete Protein Shake or two eggs to the above

- Alternatively, you may make a two egg sandwich with a little bit of cheese and whole grain bread; a small amount of bacon or sausage can also be added. You can alternatively make a breakfast burrito with a whole grain tortilla.

Finally, do not come off of this protocol and go back to your old way of eating, as doing so will make you gain the weight back, it is as simple as that. Don't waste all of the work you did by not changing your lifestyle. Follow the maintenance and healthy eating plan and you can always do the Skinny Chick! Rapid Fat Loss Protocol to lose a few pounds after vacation or holidays, etc. Do not make a habit of gaining and losing significantly though, as you will slow down your metabolism that way and it will get more and more difficult to lose weight if you yo-yo.

The good news is that it is a lot easier to maintain your weight than it is to lose it. I am an advocate for treats but my rule for myself is to eat healthy at least 90% of the time. When I do splurge, I make sure that it is something that is totally worth it and I truly enjoy it. We, as a society, revolve way too much around food and most of it is unhealthy food. Sensible diet, exercise, stress management, and finding other things besides food to live for are imperative for a healthy and long life! We are living longer than ever before but MOST people live on prescriptions and in pain and discomfort in their older years. I don't know about you but I want to live to a ripe old age and be jumping out of airplanes and hiking when I am in my seventies and eighties! Take it from a person who almost lost her life to serious illness and then got it back through living a healthy and balanced lifestyle, living with a chronic illness is no life at all! We all have a genetic propensity toward certain diseases but in most cases, our expression of those genes is completely up to us and the lifestyle we choose to live.

All too often, once somebody gets off of their weight loss diet, the trouble starts. One thing that I try very hard to make people understand is that losing weight and doing all of this work to heal your body is fantastic! You should give yourself a big pat on the back and be proud. You should not undo all of that hard work by going back to your old ways. This is where so many "diets" fall short. What do you do after your diet? Most people really have no clue how to eat a healthy, balanced diet. I know before I started studying nutrition, I did not! There is just so much information out there it confuses people. There is also way too much false advertising by food companies who are trying to pass off unhealthy foods as healthy foods. I am going to go over a plan for living that will help you maintain your fabulous weight loss, as well as a plan you can use when you are on off weeks or days, depending on how you decide to do your weight loss plan.

Let me start by saying I believe in treats... surprised? I have been known to eat the occasional hamburger, fries, (not fast food versions), chocolate, wine, etc, etc. I am nowhere near approaching overweight, so how do I do that? If you believe that you can never eat anything "bad" again if you wish to remain thin, throw that notion out the window. There is a way to eat out and splurge without gaining weight... you just have to do it correctly. My thinking is this: if you say I can never have a treat again, that is all you are going to want. If your thinking is I can have treats sometimes then you don't feel as deprived. Add to this the fact that after the weight loss portion of this diet, you are not constantly craving junk anymore and you have a real way to eat that stuff in moderation. You will have hopefully also learned a way to eat healthy that is still satisfying and tastes good so you won't feel deprived in your everyday life. I am going to further your knowledge to eat well so read on!

Tips for a Healthy Lifestyle

Eat Low on the Glycemic Index and Stay off the Sugar Roller Coaster

The glycemic index is the numerical value of how quickly a carbohydrate is broken down to glucose and put into your blood stream for use as energy by your cells or fat storage of the excess. As covered before, glucose is found in all carbohydrates and is essential for cellular energy. When any carbohydrate is eaten, the body breaks it down to its simplest cellular form, glucose, to be used by the cells for energy.

After reading Chapter 1, you have a basic understanding of how eating foods that are high in sugar or highly processed, sets you up for sugar spikes and dips that lead you to crave more sugar. This is why I call this the sugar roller coaster. A good rule of thumb is the more processed a carbohydrate is, generally the faster the sugar in it will be put into your bloodstream. Eating protein with your carbohydrates makes them break down slower, thus lowering the glycemic index. Consider this though, even if you are eating carbohydrates that are lower on the glycemic index, such as the whole grain brown rice I used as an example in chapter 1; if you eat a large amount of it and then sit on the couch for the evening, what will happen? A large portion of it will get stored as fat, as your body does not care where the glucose came from. If there is excess sugar in the system, it goes to fat storage... bottom line. Therefore, unless you are getting ready for some extreme physical activity, you will store any carbohydrate not used by the body, regardless of its source. I would like to note that if you are not in ketosis (when you are not on protocol), you do need more carbohydrates as your brain and kidneys and your body does need some carbohydrates to function. Choose the ones you do use in your daily diet wisely. I have included a glycemic index chart later on in this chapter to help you pick foods that are primarily on the lower side of the glycemic index.

What About Fruit When I am Not on the Rapid Fat Loss Protocol?

Fruit is "nature's candy" but it has many health benefits, just stick to low glycemic fruit, only eat one piece a day, and add a little protein (like almonds or unsweetened almond butter for example) to lower the glycemic index further. People often ask me why there is no fruit in the Skinny Chick! Rapid Fat Loss Protocol and the answer is simple: it is too high in sugar to allow rapid weight loss. In fact, it slows weight loss down when you are not on protocol too. That being said, especially if you are going to do harder workouts while you are off protocol or rapid loss fat times, you will need more carbohydrates and fruit is a much better option than say a highly processed snack bar for example. It is also a much more healthy option for the occasional dessert.

Are Grains an Essential Source of Nutrition?

According to the Macrobiotic diet developed by Michio Kushi, grains should be eaten as the vast majority of one's diet. This is also what the food pyramid says. Now, it is not hard to find many thousands of people who swear this diet works great for them. I, however, would not do well on this diet. When I personally consume a lot of grains, I gain weight and start having digestion and skin issues. Many, many grains are available, and many whole grains are a good source of many vitamins, minerals, protein, and fiber and can contribute to a feeling of fullness and staying full longer (in whole forms and for people who do not have issues with grains). The simple fact is that large amounts of grains can make one gain weight and cause issues, so it is wise not to consume more than you need as even whole grains break down to glucose.

There is also the issue of allergies or intolerances to certain grains. One huge offender is the gluten found in wheat, rye, barley, and oats. Some think that a large percentage of the population may be intolerant or even allergic (Celiac disease) to gluten. This can cause issues for health, as a food that one does not tolerate well cannot only wreak havoc on your body (people with celiac actually lose their villi in their small intestines, making it impossible to absorb nutrients), it can also make you either gain weight or not be able to gain weight. As with everything else, it is best to listen to your body. If you feel congested, tired, weak, and then you are hungry after you eat a certain grain or anything else for that matter, you probably don't do well on that and it may be best avoided all together.

With grains, the less processed the better, as the more processed a grain is, the higher it is on the glycemic index. Honestly, I don't think grains are an essential part of one's diet as the food pyramid claims. As far as nutrients go, they are not very much bang for your buck. You can get all of the fiber you need from fruits and veggies without all of the carbohydrates and possible health issues. My diet is very low in grains. I do have items with grains in it on occasion but stuff like that is more of an occasional treat for me and definitely not a staple. I personally avoid gluten most of the time as I suspect I have a sensitivity to it and feel better when I don't eat it on a daily basis.

Eat High in Nutrient Dense Foods

When your body is given all the nutrients it needs, we stop feeling the need to eat all the time. If we are malnourished in any way, our body will cry out for more nourishment! Unfortunately, our body won't say, 'I need more of any specific nutrient in particular', it will just cry out for more food. The more nutrient dense food you eat, the more nourished you are and the less you want to eat. Incidentally, high nutrient foods, such as most vegetables and lean proteins, are much lower in calories so you can eat more of them.

This leads me to my favorite supplement that will help your body stay very nourished with just a small amount every day… green drinks! Green drink has become almost a buzzword as of late. It makes me happy that people no longer look at me when I drink my daily green concoction and say, 'What the heck is that?!' (Well, at least less people do) like they did when I first starting drinking them eleven or so years ago. Now they often look at me and say, 'What kind do you use?'

The many ingredients, options, brands, products, and just vast array of variety and flavors can be confusing along with everything else in nutrition. This is another subject that I could write a book about all on its own so I will just cover a few key points and tell you what kind I drink. One common ingredient in many Super Food Green drinks is chlorella. This alga is a rich source of chlorophyll. It may be the best source on the planet. Chlorophyll is the richest source of a substance necessary for RNA and DNA replication in nature. I could also write a whole book on all the healthy and wonderful effects chlorophyll has on our bodies. It can help us maintain our ideal pH levels, is very detoxifying, and may be the most concentrated food per calorie on the planet in nutrients. It is important to note that you must get chlorella that has a broken cell wall (it will say broken cell wall chlorella or soft cell wall chlorella on the label), as we do not possess the enzyme to break the cellulose in the cell wall down.

Another common ingredient is spirulina, also an alga. Studies have shown it to have anti-viral and anti-cancer properties among many, many other exciting health benefits. Green drinks in general are often good sources of fiber, very bio-available protein, vitamins, minerals, and many other essential nutrients to our health. Numerous other beneficial things can be found in green drinks that are beyond the scope of this book. My favorite green drink is one called Green Vibrance by Vibrant Health, which can be purchased on Amazon.com.

Everybody I have recommended a green drink formula to has reported an increase in energy and a feeling of wellbeing. A few have even told me it was like taking a shot of espresso without the jittery feeling. I personally use Green Vibrance Green Drink instead of a vitamin supplement. I am the first to admit I have never learned to "like" the taste of green drinks; they taste like grass to me. However, I find them so essential to keep all of my nutrients high that I find ways to camouflage their taste. I add them to my Skinny Chick! Complete Protein Shakes.

What is Nutrient Negative Food?

This explanation will help you understand the proceeding sections in this chapter a bit better. A nutrient negative food is a food that takes more nutrients to digest than it actually contributes to your body. Whenever you consume anything, your body needs something to break that food down. Let's take the example of calcium and phosphorus. When you consume phosphorus, it needs calcium to be digested in a 1:1 ratio. So for every 1 phosphorus your body needs 1 calcium. Do you know where calcium is stored in your body? Your bones and teeth. So, when you drink something very high in phosphorus with no calcium (such as soda), where is your body getting the calcium it needs to break down that phosphorus? That's right... your bones and teeth.

Soda is the #1 source of calories in the United States, such a sad fact in a country where 68% of the population is overweight or obese. But why is nobody talking about another epidemic in our country... osteoporosis (weakening bone mass)? After reading the above, does it not make sense to you that since we, as a country drink a lot of soda, which is full of phosphorus and no calcium, yet needs calcium to be digested and is therefore taking it from our bones, would have a horrible bone mass or lack thereof issue? Do you ever see commercials about this? Of course not. Soda companies have a lot of money to advertise their products and drug companies have a lot of money to sell you drugs to counteract the effects that those products have on your bones, with a long list of side effects, of course. Would it not make more sense to instead educate people about drinking too much soda or phosphorus-laden foods and beverages or at least balancing your phosphorus to calcium ratio? Of course it would... but where is the profit in that?

Speaking of Soda, Don't Drink Soda

Do you have a six soda-a-day habit? Soda, pop, soft drinks, whatever you want to call them... they add zero nutrients and lots of empty calories, they are loaded with sugar, and even worse than sugar, high fructose corn syrup. I know the commercials say that high fructose corn syrup is seen by the body as sugar (which is not exactly a compliment), and they are very blasé about the health implications of it. You have to ask yourself though... who paid for that commercial? The Corn Growers Association, that's who. They obviously have everything to gain from reversing the stigma that high fructose corn syrup has and frankly deserves.

High fructose corn syrup causes an even more dramatic insulin spike than sugar. Most of it will be stored in your fat cells but even worse... your body has no idea of what to do with some of the by-products, so it will wrap them either in your fat cells or in fat globules in your liver to protect your body from harm. This is one of the many factors that leads over time to fatty liver disease, which is beyond the scope of this book to get into, but is just as bad as it sounds.

Diet sodas are far from off the hook. Besides the obvious ingredients that are possibly highly carcinogenic (cancer causing), such as aspartame, all sodas cause acidosis (an acidic state) in the body, which makes your body a perfect environment for disease and parasites to thrive. Diet soda is also very high in phosphorus, which needs calcium to be absorbed as covered above. On top of that, putting your body in an acidic state will make your body find ways to get itself back to a healthy pH level. One of the ways it will do this is by using calcium to buffer the acidity so your body will take MORE calcium from your bones to buffer the acidity. Being acidic will also make you crave sugar. So by drinking diet sodas to avoid sugar, you are setting yourself up to crave sugar later. In conclusion, regular soda consumption has no place in a healthy diet. If you want to partake in soda drinking, don't do it daily.

Eat Junk Food in Extreme Moderation or Never

As I mentioned I am a believer in treats. If we are allowed to eat certain things then we don't feel the need to gorge ourselves on them when we give into them. There are some foods however; I just won't touch, at the very least not very often. Fast food (such as big burger joint type places, McDonald's, Arby's, Wendy's and all of the others like this), as well as most of the highly processed food on store shelves, such as chips, candy bars, and all food that can sit on a shelf for years and not expire. Not only is it completely devoid of nutrients, it will steal the nutrients it needs to break down this food from the vitamins and minerals in your body, putting your body at a nutrient negative... which, as I said above, will make your body cry out for more food! In many cases, it is also harmful to your organs, as it is very difficult to break down that many artificial ingredients and, in many cases, carcinogenic ingredients. These foods are NOT worth it. After you have restored your body to a healthy state, you will most likely be repulsed by them. I know that when I even smell something like McDonald's (which used to be a staple in my diet), it makes me want to gag. Somebody sitting next to me on an airplane with it is torture!

Foods like this "dumb down" your taste buds, meaning that your taste buds are less sensitive so you need more and more salt and sugar for food to taste good. When you eat healthy food for even a few weeks, they will start to restore themselves. Food that is super sweet or salty will start to be an assault on your taste buds and they won't be tasty to you anymore. You will start to find the natural taste of natural foods appealing. This may be one of the things my clients are most skeptical about while starting out on my program but it does happen if the body is given the chance. How much easier would it be for you to make healthy choices if your body not only stopped craving so much junk food but also the healthy stuff tasted good? If you are willing to do the work to get there, you can have that. In my clinic, I find that most people want to make good choices; it is just hard when your body is crying out for junk food all the time. Even people with amazing willpower have a hard time ignoring it when their body chemically wants "bad" stuff.

Keep Healthy Food in Your House

Chopped up veggies, fruit, and cooked lean protein with good dipping sauces are ideal to keep in the house. If there is no unhealthy food to binge on in your home, you are much less likely to. I hear a lot of people say 'I always have that stuff in my house though because my kids eat it.' My answer to that is 'kids don't get the food, the parents do.' If they are snacking on junk food, they will have the lifelong struggle with weight and disease that most Americans do. Do you want your children to struggle with this, just as you are now? Educate your children about food and help them create healthy lifestyle habits so they don't have to struggle with it later.

I am currently creating a nutrition program for children book, as I have been very successful in finding ways to help children understand and care about nutrition in my clinic. The best way, if it is not too late already to get kids to eat healthy, is to start them out that way and eat healthy in front of them. When they are young and impressionable, they won't know any better and they will likely want whatever you are having. My little girl did not know anything but healthy food until other people started giving unhealthy food to her. She ate whole foods and occasional treats and that was completely normal to her. It is harder for me to control that now that she is in school but she actually likes her chicken and cauliflower or broccoli and all the other healthy options I give her.

Here is a story that is a serious reflection of the society we live in as it pertains to food. I took my daughter to her first day at a new pre-school; she was four at the time. As she was walking us to the classroom, the teacher said, "We have a guinea pig named Oreo... can you guess what color he is?" My daughter thought about it for a second and then shouted out, "Orange!" The teacher looked at me like, what is wrong with this kid?! I explained that mom is a nutritionist and that my child had never had an Oreo or obviously ever even seen one. She thought that was crazy.

Another story... a big group of new friends could not believe that my five year old had never had a soda in her life. We were at a wedding and I let my daughter order a Shirley Temple as a treat since we were all having some wine and she wanted something special. She freaked out the first time carbonation hit her tongue, she didn't like it, and she had never experienced it before. My friends took that as proof she had never had soda and believed me; however, they could not believe it because it is so unusual for a five year old never to have had soda. I have a lot more stories like this. I am often perceived as weird for not raising my child on junk food. This notion is crazy to me: I don't think it is that people think it is a bad thing for the most part, many people simply can't believe I have managed to raise my child this way. This is the way our family lives; this is all she knows and she does not find it strange at all. I educate her and even at the age of seven, she knows more about nutrition than most adults do. I do not consider that a bad thing or myself strange for raising her this way. I would very much like to contribute to the end of the attitude that all people should be aware of what Oreos and sodas are and should consume them frequently, as well as the attitude that any child who doesn't consume these has "crazy" parents.

Fat, Possibly the Most Misunderstood Nutrient There is

I went over this briefly in the Skinny Chick! Rapid Fat Loss Protocol chapter. This will stay true in maintenance. Not only is fat essential for your weight loss goals, it is also essential for the absorption of several nutrients. I encourage you to do your own research on this subject.

Plan Ahead, Keep Your Body Fueled, and Listen to Your Body

Eating healthy is about planning ahead and staying ahead of your hunger. If you get to the point where you are "starving", you will most likely not crave a healthy option, you will most likely crave an unhealthy one. If you keep your body fueled with healthy food and stay ahead of your hunger, you will be much more able to stay in control. Listen to your body. If something makes your energy suddenly bottom out, there is something going on. It could be a food intolerance, or your body could just not like that food at that time of the day. I don't do well on carbohydrates in the morning, as they make my pulse speed up and then I crave carbohydrates all day if I eat them too early. Get in tune with your body, and you will start to figure out the way your body works best... all you have to do is pay attention.

Then What Should I Eat?

We covered a lot of what not to eat didn't we? So what should you eat? Well, my normal diet looks like the protocol diet only with some stuff added, such as vegetables that are not included on the protocol due to their higher carbohydrate content, some fruit, and some treats thrown in here and there.

I get the question a lot, so here it is... no, I do not eat "perfectly". When I first got really into health and nutrition, I did. I was obsessed with everything I put in my body to the point that I could not go out to eat with my friends because there was never anything pure or healthy enough to eat where they went. I have been through many, many phases in my journey to health and honestly, my opinions and approaches are still constantly evolving, as I am still constantly learning new things.

What then constitutes a healthy diet? Eating a variety of healthy foods, absolutely. Keep it in perspective though. Life is so much more than food. I know that sounds so silly to even say but I have lived through not being able to do anything for fear of eating something slightly unhealthy. This is no way to live; I have balanced out now. When I go to a friend's house that has put in a great deal of effort to make me a lovely meal, I will not sit at their table and refuse to eat something because I know it is not healthy. I still even have the occasional well-meaning person who makes me a cake for my birthday not knowing that I hate cake (yes, HATE it, way too sweet!) and I will choke some of that down because if somebody cared enough to make me some cake then I will eat some and pretend to like it. If I go to a restaurant with my friends and they are known for their amazing burgers and fries, I will order a burger and fries. I will not eat the whole burger, I will cut it in half, and I will most likely eat way too many fries, as they are one of my favorite treats. The next day, I will go right back to my normal, healthy lifestyle.

I am to the point where my normal diet that consists mostly of my protein shakes with my green drink added, large salads, vegetables, eggs, animal proteins, nuts, some yogurt, some natural cheese, lots of healthy fats (40% plus of my diet is fat), fruit, and the occasional dark, natural chocolate, and other treats and wine thrown in appeals to me. Long gone are the days of pasta, bread, and rice being a staple for me, as well as always including rolls or some kind of carbohydrate at dinner. I would say my staple now is vegetables, which is why I have come up with so many different recipes and variations to cook them in, as I share in Chapter 9. When I stray too far from this norm, such as over the holidays and on vacation; I miss it and how great I feel when I am loving myself by eating healthy and working out. You can get to this point too.

I still employ my Skinny Chick! Rapid Fat Loss Protocol after a particularly bad cheat day, after vacation, or after the holiday season, to help avoid storing fat, to reset, and knock myself out of the pattern of picking unhealthy food, and sometimes to lose a few pounds. Being healthy, fit, and in the body you want to be in is completely addictive. I never want to go back to the old me... and you won't either! Starting below is a glycemic index chart for a lot of common carbohydrate foods. Eat low on the glycemic index as often as possible and stay off the sugar roller coaster! This is also one of the helpful tools you can download in a printable version at skinnychickweightloss.com

Glycemic Index Food Chart

The majority of your diet should be in the 55 or lower range with the majority of that being in the 30 and below range. This is especially true if you are already pre-diabetic or have type 2 diabetes.

30 and Below - Low

30-55 - Medium

55-70 - High

70 and Above - Very High

<u>**Vegetables**</u>	
Artichoke	15
Asparagus	15
Broccoli	15
Cauliflower	15
Celery	15
Cucumber	15
Eggplant	15
Lettuce, all varieties	15
Snow peas	15
Spinach	15
Young summer squash	15
Zucchini	15

Soy beans, boiled	16
Peppers, all varieties	20
Green beans	20
Peas	22
Carrots	39
Parsnips	52
Beets	59
Sweet Corn	60
Potatoes	
Yam	51
Sweet potato	54
Potato, boiled	56
Potato, steamed	65
Potato, mashed	70
Potato Chips	75
Potato, microwaved	82
Potato, instant	83
Potato, baked	85
Fruit	
Avocado	15
Cherries	22
Grapefruit	25

Strawberries/Blackberries/ Raspberries/Blueberries	32
Apples	38
Pears	38
Tomatoes	38
Plums	39
Peaches	42
Oranges	44
Grapes	46
Kiwi fruit	53
Bananas	54
Fruit cocktail (no added sugar)	55
Mangoes	56
Apricots	57
Apricots (tinned in syrup)	64
Raisins	64
Cantaloupe	65
Pineapple	66
Watermelon	72
Dates (dried)	90
Beans	
Kidney beans, boiled	29
Lentils green, boiled	29

Black Beans	29
Chickpeas	33
Black-eyed peas	41
Baked beans	48
Refried Beans	55
Dairy Foods	
Yogurt (unsweetened)	14
Milk, whole	27
Milk, Fat-free	32
Milk, skimmed	34
Ice-cream	61
Beverages	
Soy milk	30
Wine (dry no sugar added)	0-20
Hard Liquor (no sugar added)	0-20
Apple juice	41
Vegetable Juice (tomato based)	44
Pineapple juice	46
Grapefruit juice	48

Orange juice	52
Beer	73
Carrot juice	77
Grains and Bread	
Pearl barley	25
Rice, brown non-instant	25
Rye	34
Rice, wild	40
Wheat kernels	41
Quinoa	45
Rice, instant	46
Multi grain bread	48
Whole grain	50
Barley, cracked	50
Rice, brown instant	55
Pita bread, white	57
Rice, white	58
Pizza, cheese	60
Popcorn	60
Hamburger bun	61
Muffin (unsweetened)	62
Rye-flour bread	64
Barley, flakes	66

Croissant	67
Taco Shell	68
Whole meal bread	69
White bread	71
Millet	71
Bagel (plain)	72
Saltines	72
White rolls	73
Rice cakes	77
Waffles/pancakes	77
Stuffing	77
Baguette	95
Breakfast Cereals	
Oatmeal steel cut, unsweetened	38
All-Bran	42
Porridge, non-instant	49
Oat bran	55
Muesli	56
Mini Wheats (unsweetened)	57
Shredded Wheat	69
Golden Grahams	71
Puffed wheat	74

Oatmeal Instant	75
Cheerios (unsweetened)	75
Rice Krispies	82
Cornflakes	83
Pasta	
Spaghetti, protein enriched	27
Fettuccine	32
Vermicelli	35
Spaghetti, whole wheat	37
Ravioli, meat filled	39
Spaghetti, white	41
Macaroni	45
Spaghetti, durum wheat	55
Macaroni and cheese	64
Rice pasta	92
Sweeteners	
Stevia	0-0.5
Agave	15
Brown Rice Syrup	25
Raw honey	30
Maple Syrup	54
Evaporated Cane Juice	55

Black Strap Molasses	55
Brown Sugar	64
Table sugar (sucrose)	100
High Fructose Corn Syrup	102
Miscellaneous Junk Food	
Danish pastry	59
Cake , tart	65
Cake, angel	67
Corn chips	74
Doughnut	76
Vanilla wafers	77
Jelly beans	80
Pretzels	81
Cake, Chocolate and vanilla	80-90
Most Candy	80–95

Chapter 5
The Case for Organic

No discussion about nutrition is complete without discussing organic. I get questions about it often and find it to be a widely misunderstood subject. This subject is a BIG one and I would have to make this book very long indeed to even come close to approaching the tip of the iceberg so this will just be more of a basic, very brief crash course on why anybody would choose these foods. Everybody has at least heard the term organic as it pertains to food in their lives. People assume that anything that is labeled organic is automatically healthy even if it is something like organic toaster pastries. Just because something is labeled organic does not necessarily make it healthy. The USDA (United States Department of Agriculture) designation of certified organic means that all of the ingredients in the product have been proven to be free of pesticides, artificial additives, artificial preservatives, hormones, antibiotics, and several other potentially harmful ingredients. All farmers certified under this seal must also use sustainable means of farming and are visited by FDA inspectors to ensure compliance. For more information on USDA organic designation, please visit www.ams.usda.gov/nop/.

Many see the prices of organic products and turn away not knowing the value organic food may provide. So what exactly are the reasons that we keep hearing we should eat organic? The following are some of the known reasons to choose organic whenever possible. Please be aware that this list is only the tip of the iceberg and meant for general information. Even if it were possible for me to give you a pamphlet with all the known information on all the different aspects that go into making nonorganic food (it would take forever to read), there are certainly still undiscovered consequences to all the various things that we have done to our food, water, air, and earth in general.

Pesticides

Let's start with pesticides, herbicides, etc. There are so many pesticides, herbicides, and other artificial chemicals that either have been or are in use in modern agriculture that it would be ridiculous to list them all and what each particular one is known to do. In general, pesticides and other artificial chemicals are used on nonorganic produce to rid crops of all pests... as the name pesticides implies. They generally do this by killing the pests by shutting down their central nervous system. According to Patrick Holford, founder of The Institute of Optimum Nutrition and author of *The New Optimum Nutrition Bible* cited at the end, the average person eats around a gallon of pesticides on their fruits and vegetables alone in the course of a year.

The first type of pesticides widely used for agriculture were called organochlorines. These proved to be so toxic and non-biodegradable that they were eventually banished in many parts of the world, including the United States. They were then replaced by organaophosphates, which are now widely used in the United States. Some of the issues found to have a possible link to these types of pesticides include carcinogenic properties, implicated in causing birth defects and infertility, and can be very toxic to the brain and nervous system in general. Exposure has also been linked to depression, memory decline, aggression, and Parkinson's disease. That is just an incomplete list of the effects that are suspected. Nobody knows how these things may react with any of the other endless list of artificial chemicals commonly found in our food supply and what issues that may cause.

Aside from hurting our bodies directly via our food, all the runoff from these operations that use such chemicals ends up in our water supply, which we drink, all fish swim in, and animals drink, and we all accumulate these substances in our tissues. So, there is no way to even estimate just how much of these compounds we are ingesting and what they are doing to us. Pesticides also degrade the soil of its minerals and nutrients, thus making the produce grown on that land less and less full of these with every passing year of artificial chemical use. Several studies indicate that organic produce not only tastes better, but that it also provides many more nutrients than conventionally grown produce. This makes sense now doesn't it?

Another issue is Genetically Modified foods, also known as GMO foods. One way GMO foods are created is by genetically engineering crops (big offenders are corn and soy) to be resistant to herbicides so crops can be sprayed with herbicides, indiscriminately killing all the weeds with little work thus improving crop yield and cutting back on worker pay; in other words, increasing profit. Manufacturers have created ways to make crops more drought resistant through genetic modification, and many plants that produce their own compounds that are deadly to insects. Some proponents of GMO products claim that these products are completely safe for human consumption and that this scientific breakthrough will make it much more possible to feed the masses while greatly increasing profit for the growers.

The truth is that the consequences of these methods for food production are not yet known. All the things known about GMO foods are beyond the scope of this book. It is an issue I feel everybody should educate themselves on. What we know is that despite the fact that GMO foods are supposed to lessen the need for pesticides and herbicides, more of both are in use than ever before, much more. We also know that these species tend to "invade" all surrounding crops and spread. There have been cases of organic farmers who discovered GMO strains in their crops that had spread from a neighboring crop. This not only means that they lose their USDA organic seal due to the fact that GMO foods are prohibited under this umbrella; it also means that since these GMO strains are patented and can only be used if purchased, organic farmers can and do get sued for having these strains spread to their crops. Sadly, the large corporations with their vast wealth suing the small farmers, often win.

The known reactions so far to this new trend where health is concerned are antibiotic resistance, creation of new toxins, and many known allergic reactions to these foods. There is also some preliminary concern that these methods used to get produce to express or wake up certain genes to produce different or more resilient crops, may be "waking up" unwanted gene expressions in the humans consuming them.

One example I often think of when it comes to messing with nature in this way is Killer Bees. Killer Bees were created when Brazilian scientists took some African Bees to Brazil to try to create a bee that would be more able to handle living in tropical areas. Some of the bees escaped and started breeding with local Brazilian bees. This eventually led to an Africanized Honey Bee, which is a crossbreed of the Brazilian and African Bees, to start emerging and creating colonies. These bees are incredibly aggressive and were dubbed killer bees due to the fact that they will viscously attack and kill any animal or person who inadvertently wanders into their territory. They are a serious menace and are circling the globe at an alarming rate… all because the Brazilian scientists wanted better honey. It seems that no matter how many lessons we find in nature to elude that it is best to leave it alone, the human race does not seem to heed the warning. Speaking of bees, honeybees are also at a serious threat of being killed out by pesticides. Do you like fruit and flowers? Without bees to pollinate, we can say goodbye to them. The only way presently to avoid GMO foods or pesticides in your food is to eat organic.

Pesticides in our food and GMO foods are just two cases related to organic versus nonorganic, which involves whole foods, such as fruits or vegetables. Many thousands of artificial colorings, artificial chemicals, artificial preservatives, etc. are used in processed foods. The complexity of this issue is far beyond the scope of this book as there are just too many artificial chemicals to mention. There are currently approximately 3000 plus artificial chemical food additives used in foods in the United States today. It is estimated that the average American consumes up to one-hundred-and-fifty to sixty pounds of food additives each year. These additives have been proven to cause such a wide range of issues that they can't all be covered here but include carcinogenic, nervous system damage, gene mutations, toxicity issues, behavioral issues, aggression issues, organ and tissue damage, fertility issues... the list goes on and on. I personally am more concerned about all the implications for the way we manufacture food that have not been discovered yet. The fact is that we just don't know how much damage we have done and are doing to our planet and our bodies.

Hormones and Antibiotics

Hormones and antibiotics are routinely added to all commercial animals and therefore are in all commercial animal products. Remember how I explained to you that your body takes any toxins it can't get rid of via normal means and stores them in your fat cells? Animal's bodies do the same thing. Hormones are injected into animals to boost production by making them grow as fat and as fast as possible, as well as to make them produce more milk. All the added hormones have been implicated in the fact that young people are now hitting puberty much earlier than they ever have. It is also thought to be one of the reasons that women are going through menopause earlier and that there is such a surge of hormone related cancers, such as breast and uterine cancers.

Antibiotics are used routinely in the food of the feedlot animals due to the fact that the conditions of these places are so crowded, filthy, stressful, and inhumane to the animals that they need them to control disease outbreaks and infections. The overuse of antibiotics is a huge factor in antibiotic resistant strains of bacteria so prevalent today. It is also known that antibiotics wipe out all of the good flora in the gut, making individuals much more susceptible to various parasites and other pathogens. Unbalanced gut flora also leads to a seriously compromised ability to absorb nutrients and digest foods properly, setting the body up for serious digestion issues, including Diverticulitis, Irritable Bowel Disease, Irritable Bowel Syndrome, and many other ailments, and as it pertains to this book, weight gain.

Animal Cruelty

Of course, no discussion on organic principles can be complete without the mention of animal cruelty. The places where conventionally grown animals are raised for slaughter are not even called farms anymore. They are called feedlots. These places are so disgusting, toxic, and awful that I will not mention many of the details of how these places run here but will instead include references to books for further reading. This is because so many people find the things that happen to the animals in these feedlots so disturbing that they get incredibly angry at me for telling them. I am sure the small amount I know of it from a philosophy class I took on the subject in college is not even close to all of it but again, it is much too lengthy to list here.

One thing I will mention is that the toxins, pollutants, pathogens, and other things we don't even know about yet found in the vast amounts of manure from these feedlots are the number one contributor to the pollution of our air and waterways... number one, that is not a typo. As if that is not enough, the inhumane atrocities committed to these animals should be criminal in my opinion. I believe that awareness is key and that most people would care deeply about what goes on in these factories of torture if they only knew. I urge you to educate yourself on this issue even though it is very disturbing, and I have included some excellent books to get you started at the end of this chapter.

Why does the government and the world for that matter allow our world and our bodies to be polluted with chemicals and our animals to be exploited, abused, and tortured? There is a simple answer to this: money and ignorance. Money on the part of the industry that enjoys very large profits at the expense of our planet, us, our animals, and the world. Money on the part of the government officials who allow these things to go on and are rewarded political contributions and often jobs at various chemical, pharmaceutical, and food giants when they leave office. Ignorance on the part of the public, not in a way of stupidity but just that most people can't imagine, can't believe that our U.S. government and people in general would do or allow this. What can we do? Buy organic, it is as simple as that. Organic is more expensive but as more and more people buy organic, the demand for it will go up and thus the supply and the cost will drop. I think it can be argued that the only way to stop these giant food industries from conducting business as usual is to hit them where it will hurt them: their pocket books. We can appeal to the feedlot owners, the large corporations and the government. That will certainly raise awareness but they are clearly just fine with the status quo. If we stop buying their products on a large enough scale, they will be forced to adhere to better guidelines so that we may consider buying their products again. One person really can make a difference. This has already been happening in the last ten years on a large scale, as I have seen the availability and affordability of many organic foods go way up! This is good news… the food industry is listening.

If you can't afford to eat exclusively organic food, that is understandable. It is more expensive to eat exclusively organic, there is no denying that. The most important product to buy organic is animal products. The fact that you are getting so much nasty stuff in the animals you eat from the disgusting and unnatural way most conventional animals are raised is reason enough to do your best to switch animal products to organic as much as possible. The higher fat content of a conventionally raised animal, the more disgusting things you are ingesting. Items, such as butter and high fat content meats, would be a good place to start to switch to organic. As far as all the organic processed foods on the market now, are they better than conventional? Without a doubt… yes! However, even organic super refined foods need to be limited. If you eat an organic toaster pastry, you will not be ingesting GMO ingredients or pesticides but you will still be eating too high on the glycemic index. Organic junk food is still junk food.

There is a list called the "Dirty Dozen", which is a list of the most contaminated produce. Look at this list below if you need a place to start for choosing which produce to buy organic.

The Dirty Dozen

- Apples
- Strawberries
- Grapes
- Celery
- Peaches
- Spinach
- Sweet bell peppers
- Nectarines (imported)
- Cucumbers
- Cherry tomatoes
- Snap peas (imported)
- Potatoes

Further Reading and Resources

www.ams.usda.gov/nop/

<u>Staying Healthy with Nutrition</u> by Elson M. Hass MD (a lot of information on chemicals and what ailments individual ones are known to cause)

<u>The Omnivore's Dilemma</u> by Michael Pollan (a lot of information on animal cruelty, modern agricultural practices, the history of agriculture and how we got here as well as a lot of information on GMO food and animal feed lots, behind the scenes)

<u>Harvest for Hope</u> by Jane Goodall (a lot of information on animal cruelty and what we can do to put a stop to it)

<u>Food, Inc.</u> The movie (explanation of where our food comes from)

*I have no affiliation and receive no monetary gain from these sights or recommendations. This is for informational purposes only. It is not my intent to diagnose or cure any disease.

Chapter 6
Measuring to Track Results and Plateaus

It is important to keep track of your results. I keep track of my clients' results by using a combination of body measurements and weight on a fancy scale that tracks your fat percentage, water percentage, and muscle percentage so I can make sure those numbers are remaining on track. I am starting to love before and after pictures too though. The reason is that when you hit the inevitable plateau and start to get discouraged, it can be helpful to take a new picture and look back to where you started while you get through it. Although I do still work one-on-one with some clients, it is not practical or even possible to work with everybody who will read this book. So I will walk you through how and when to do these measurements at home with help or on your own so you can watch your body change. I really encourage you to do this, as watching the results as they happen can really keep you motivated!

Weighing In

Let's start with weighing yourself as it is the most obvious way to track weight loss. As I said, I use a fancy scale that measures fat percentage, muscle percentage, and water percentage among other measurements. This is useful for many reasons if you can afford to purchase one. Search fat loss scales on Amazon.com and you will get a lot of options and price ranges. I use a pretty fancy Tanita brand scale that the average person cannot afford for home use and it is pretty accurate, but you can get decent fat loss scales that are not expensive.

This is useful because seeing what is happening on the inside is often more encouraging for clients. The reason is that fat is dense and not heavy. With typical diets, you lose mostly muscle and water weight, which might show a bigger loss on the scale, but won't change the body composition as much as most people would like. Think of it this way, muscle is twice as heavy as fat because it is much denser taking up half the space that fat does in your body. Since you will be losing mostly fat percentage, you might be showing more weight loss in different ways (such as body measurements and in how your clothing fits) than you will on the scale. Don't get me wrong, you will still show significant loss on the scale. I just want you to understand that you may lose more in other ways. If you are also going to be working out and consuming Skinny Chick! Complete Protein Shakes, helping you gain muscle mass, you will start looking so different, but you may not be satisfied with what the scale says.

Cutting carbohydrates can also cause water retention in some people, which is the biggest discouraging factor for my clients. With a scale that breaks these things down for you, it is easier to see what is going on inside of your body. Keep in mind though that these scales are not 100% accurate. One thing that can drive me crazy with these scales is the fact that sometimes when people get water logged; the fat percentage will suddenly jump up when my clients have been doing everything correctly. Once I get them on my Skinny Chick! Bloat Eraser supplement for a few days, the fat percentage and water percentage usually drops back down.

Another thing to keep in mind with weighing yourself is do not weigh yourself multiple times a day or even every day. Our weight fluctuates a lot throughout the day! Think about all the water and food you consume throughout the day; it has an effect on your weight. In fact, if you drink a huge glass of water and then hop on a fat percentage scale, it will usually show a rapid fat percentage increase. Do not do this to yourself, as you will drive yourself insane. I challenge my clients that I work one-on-one with to not weigh themselves at home and only weigh in on their weekly visits with me on my scale. I also try to book clients once a week at basically the same time. For you, the reader doing this at home, pick a day to weigh yourself once a week and first thing in the morning. People tend to splurge a little more than usual over the weekend so do not pick Monday. For most people, a good morning will be Thursday or Friday morning when you have been adhering to your healthy ways all week perfectly and you should be retaining the least amount of water.

Honestly, scales drive me a bit insane. I watch my clients become obsessed with the number on those scales because that is what we have been taught. I own three fancy scales that I get on maybe twice a year, yep, only twice a year. The reason is this: I go by how I feel and how my clothing feels. When I work out heavily that number may go up due to increasing my muscle mass (which is a very good thing, and we will get to that in the next chapter). I am simply not obsessed with what my number on the scale is because I would rather have a lot of lean muscle mass, low fat mass, and a higher number on the scale than a low number on the scale while not having the shape I want.

Measuring To Watch the Inches Fall Off

Measuring yourself is a very good way to keep track of your fat loss. My clients are often most impressed with the inch loss, which is usually quite significant. I do quite a few measurements with my clients that will not be possible to do on yourself but the following are some instructions for how to measure yourself at home to track your inch loss. It is important to wear the same type of clothing when you measure or measure your bare skin. Do your best to measure in the same spot, as well as with the tape measure at the same tightness each time you do measure. A measurement chart is included with the free downloads at skinnychickweightloss.com. Use a measuring tape, such as the ones you use for fabric. Measurements are best done once a week in the morning. With my clients, I do them at the same time as weigh in.

Bust Measurement

Measure with the tape around your bust and across the middle of your nipples. Make sure that the tape does not bow down in the back. Wear the same bra every time you measure, as different bras make a big difference in measurements.

Waist Measurement

Measure with the tape around the belly and meeting in the middle of the belly button while trying to ensure the tape does not bow down in the back.

Hip Measurement

Measure with the tape around the hips and resting over the pointy part of your hipbone. For some people, it makes more sense to measure lower on the butt if that is a spot they would like to lose. Just be certain that you are measuring approximately the same spot every time.

Thigh Measurement

Measure with the tape from the top inside of your thigh down to a spot on your inner thigh that you are comfortable measuring around. Write how far you measured down your inner thigh on your measurement chart so that you can attempt to get roughly the same spot every time. Stick to one thigh or measure both, and don't measure different thighs each time you measure.

Arm Measurement

This measurement will be very difficult to do on your own; if you can get somebody else to do this for you, it will be much easier. Measure with the tape from the outside edge of your armpit to about four or five inches down your arm depending on the length of your arm. Mark this point with your finger and then take the tape around the arm to get the measurement.

Before and After Photos

Before and after photos can be invaluable in your weight loss journey. As I said before, they can make you feel better when you hit a plateau so you can see how far you have come and not get discouraged. Do one picture from the front and one from the side. Take pictures just before you start and then at least at the end to see the amazing transformation for yourself. I do not recommend taking pictures more than once a week, as not seeing a change every single day may be discouraging for some. If you would like to help inspire others by sharing your before and after photos on my website, please visit www.completeweightlossandwellness.com and contact me to discuss it. Testimonials and before and after photos go a long way toward helping others decide to take the leap into changing their unhealthy habits.

I do believe that the best way to track your progress is to see how you feel. I especially always notice a difference in my clothing. I have one pair of skinny jeans that are my marker.

If I don't fit in those comfortably anymore (such as after the holidays or after vacation), I know it is time to get myself in check. I also have people point out areas that we did not measure that have improved dramatically, such as the saggy stuff right on top of your bra or under your bra. Pay attention to these things as watching that improve is encouraging.

Plateaus

My least favorite and most unavoidable issue with my clients: plateaus. Plateaus happen to 98% of the people that I work with so the likelihood that it will happen at least once to you is high. I have heard a weight loss plateau defined as any span of three weeks during which a person does not lose weight but for my clients, I consider one week without any loss a plateau. I really don't want anybody getting to a three-week plateau, but it does happen every once in a great while. What I try to tell people is this: our bodies do not want to let go of extra weight; they want to hold onto that weight in case we experience famine.

When you hit a plateau that means your body has gotten to a new place of comfort… smaller than where you started. Remember how I told you that maintaining your weight is far easier than losing weight, well in a plateau, you now have your body to this new place of "normal" that will be easy to maintain. If you have not reached your goal, it is understandable that you want to push through that new point of comfort to an even lower point of comfort. The good news is that this can be done.

To break through a plateau, you need to shake it up somehow and re-shock your body into losing again. If you do the same thing to your body over and over, it does adjust to this as the new normal and your fat loss can slow down. One way to push through a plateau is to simply take a thermogenic, which is a supplement that accelerates fat loss. I sell an excellent one in my Amazon.com store that includes all of the big and very popular fat acceleration supplements, such as Garcinia Cambogia and green tea extract plus much more in one called Skinny Chick! Thermo. If you have been on the Skinny Chick! Rapid Fat Loss portion of the plan for an extended period of time, get into maintenance for at least a week and take a break. I have a lot of people who strongly resist this approach and think I am insane for suggesting it, but it does help to take a break from it. Taking a break can help your body respond better to the rapid fat loss portion when you start again. Yet another thing you can do is change up your workout. If you are not going for a nice, brisk walk every day, maybe now is the time to start. Simply changing something up is sometimes all it takes to break through the plateau quickly!

Another issue that some people have is that they have simply become too acidic. This can happen for a variety of reasons. For example, I definitely find this to be the case with people who refuse to give up their diet sodas or alcohol. The acidity of the soda and alcohol plus the added acidity of your body turning fat into ketones to use as energy just pushes them past the acidity threshold. If your body becomes too acidic, your fat loss will stop, and your body will start focusing on bringing your pH level back to a healthy range. People can use supplements that specifically work on creating a healthy pH to help break through it faster. If you are going to stop the rapid fat loss protocol for a week and do a week of maintenance, a very good supplement is Green Vibrance, which is a green, super food mix that I suggest you put in your protein shake. It can be purchased at many health food stores, such as Whole Foods, but is much less expensive on Amazon.com. There is also a myriad of pH lowering drops on the market that you add to your drinking water that do the trick for many of my clients. Please check out Chapter 8 for details and where to purchase them.

In the midst of a plateau, it is important to keep in mind that it will eventually pass, that it happens to almost everybody, and is a normal part of weight loss. I very often see people have a huge drop in their weight and fat percentage at the conclusion of a plateau. Your body is still doing a lot of amazing work even if you are not seeing your numbers budge from the outside. Try to be grateful that your body has a new comfort set point that is lower than where you started.

One more thing to keep in mind in weight loss is that the lower your weight gets and the closer you get to your goal, the more your loss will slow down. This is more difficult for my clients who started out with a lot of excess weight, as some of these clients lose large amounts of weight initially. This is normal and to be expected. However, the closer you get to your goal, the lower amount of fat loss it will take to see big differences! If you only have ten pounds to go, two pounds will be noticeable, for example.

Chapter 7
Working Out During Protocol and on Maintenance

No discussion about weight loss is complete without a discussion about working out. Working out is an excellent way to lose and maintain your new lower weight. The mistake I see most often with clients who have come to me for help when they worked out hard and saw little to no results with their weight loss from it is that they were not working out correctly for fat loss and that they were not eating correctly for fat loss while they were working out. I am all about doing things in the easiest way possible. I don't know about you but I do not want to feel like a gerbil on a wheel running on a treadmill for an hour a day and get little result from it. I have gone to great lengths to research how to get the most bang for my workout buck and I will pass that on to you.

Let's discuss working out while on protocol before we go any further. Working out hard while on protocol WILL slow your weight loss down. I am not saying it is impossible to do it... I am saying that if you want to maximize your rapid fat loss weeks, do not work out to excess. I have had client after client after client test me on this, and I am always proven correct. Doing lighter workouts, such as walking, yoga, and some light weight lifting, is perfect for rapid fat loss protocol weeks. Save the heavy workouts for the weeks you take off from the rapid fat loss protocol. If you are a big workout buff and you enjoy your hard workouts, consider doing rapid fat loss protocol and light workouts one week and maintenance plus heavy workout weeks every other week. This will ensure that you still get your heavy workouts that will build nice lean muscle for you and you will get both a week of rapid fat and toxin dumping plus a week of rest for your muscles to regenerate, which is equally important to getting in good physical condition.

The most important thing to exercise is finding a workout you can enjoy. I do not enjoy running for hours on end but some people do enjoy that. Find what works for you! There are SO many choices out there in workouts. One thing that is wise to incorporate is some kind of muscle work. The reason is that building lean muscle will turn your body into a fat burning machine. The more muscle you have, the more your body burns calories and fat at all times. This is one of the many reasons that men lose weight so much easier than women do in general. I find a lot of women are afraid to gain too much muscle. Honestly though, that is very difficult to do for most women. What will happen most likely is that you will end up with a very sleek and toned look, which in my opinion, is a healthy look and one I certainly strive for.

Let's talk cardio. I do find most people think that doing long cardio workouts is the way to weight loss. I personally do not have two hours a day to devote to exercise, but if you do, good on you! However, as I said, I like to find the best bang for my workout buck! I have come across something called Peak Fitness coined by Dr. Mercola. With peak fitness, you push it as hard as you can for about thirty seconds and recover for about ninety seconds. You repeat this process for a total of around eight repetitions that you can do in roughly twenty minutes. When I changed my cardio from long, drawn out cardio sessions that I had to drag myself through to this type of training, I personally saw a huge increase in my fat loss and fitness level. This also gave me more time for muscle building, which I of course find so important. Google Peak Fitness and read up. I find it to be the second best discovery I have ever made in working out. When I am done with this regimen, I am energized, sweaty, and definitely on that exercise endorphin high that can make workouts addictive (again, not a bad thing to be addicted to). I know it is unbelievable to imagine that you can get so much out of twenty minutes (I do more like twenty-five minutes with a longer warm up and cool down) but I have found it to absolutely be the case.

The best discovery I have ever made in amping up my work out and getting the most out of it is how to eat around it. This method applies mostly to people who are doing a moderate amount of exercise as opposed people who are training for a marathon or any kind of high energy output type of sport. I work out early in the morning, as this is the time of day that works best for me; it also gets me energized and ready for the day and gets it out of the way and done. I work out on an empty stomach if I start early enough; if not, I have something with some carbohydrates, such as a small piece of fruit or a low sugar yogurt, to get me through my work out without a tank in energy. I believe the big key to getting the most out of your fat burn is what you do after your workout.

When you work out hard and get your heart rate up, you ignite something called an HGH (Human Growth Hormone) surge. Peak Fitness is an excellent way to attain this surge. HGH production has been shown to decrease with age. There has been a gain in popularity with people injecting HGH for fitness and beauty, but I do not recommend this. A lot of side effects to this approach are undesirable and unhealthy and well beyond the scope of this small chapter on working out. Let's just say it backfires, and people are finding they actually age faster with this very unnatural approach to an HGH surge.

A natural, cheap, and easy way is to simply do a very good, strenuous workout followed up with proper nutrition. This can include perhaps some muscle work with weights, and then Peak Fitness exercise followed up by taking a Skinny Chick! Complete Protein Shake. One of the biggest mistakes I see people continuing to make after a hard workout is eating something with a lot of carbohydrates. Eating let's say a piece of fruit, which I find to be a popular workout recovery item among my clients, a recovery shake that contains a lot of sugar and or carbohydrates, or a sugary sport drink does one thing to you: it stops your HGH surge. You want this HGH surge to happen, as this is part of what builds muscle, burns fat, and keeps you aging slowly. Having a whey protein isolate shake, such as the Skinny Chick! Complete Protein Shake, will not only replenish you after a hard workout, but it does not contain the sugar and fast carbohydrates that will kill your HGH burn. As an added bonus, whey protein isolate has been shown to not only help you build muscle but it can also help increase your HGH production post workout. By also adding a scoop of L-Glutamine powder to your recovery shake, you can speed up the muscle recovery process. My husband and I use Now brand L-Glutamine powder in our recovery shakes.

One of the great things my Skinny Chick! Rapid Fat Loss Protocol can achieve is in helping your body regain a healthy insulin and leptin sensitivity and reverse insulin resistance. Adding the correct workouts to this will help greatly in speeding this process up and enhancing it. If you can regain healthy insulin and leptin resistance, which by the way is completely attainable for anybody. You can get to a point where your body has a normal, healthy response to carbohydrates, which is one of the ultimate goals of this program. If you are new to working out, start slowly so that you do not injure yourself and give yourself the time and patience to ease into it slowly. Also, keep in mind that working out too much can be a bad thing. If you do too much, especially too soon and do not give your muscles proper time for recovery, you will slow your weight loss down, as your body will want to conserve energy and will be focused on recovery. Investing in a certified personal trainer to learn proper workout form, methods, and skills at least once is a good investment in yourself if you can afford it.

Most of all, try to enjoy it. Working out like anything else is all about perspective. I have a rule for myself that when I really don't feel like working out, I resolve to do it for at least fifteen minutes. Ninety eight percent of the time, after fifteen minutes it starts to feel good for me and I want to keep going. I also shake it up. I love doing dance type workouts like Zumba and I have quite the collection of workout videos to choose from. I also really enjoy taking classes such as Zumba and kickboxing to work out with others. If I get sick of it and I no longer look forward to doing it, I move onto something else. Above all, I want to enjoy my workout and feel amazing, strong, and powerful when I am done.

Chapter 8
Supplements and Supplement Instructions

As I mentioned in Chapter 2, some supplements are required to do this protocol safely. We will start with these supplements and elaborate on how to take them. All Skinny Chick! brand supplements can be purchased at Amazon.com

Required Supplements

Skinny Chick! Complete Protein Shake

We already covered this extensively in Chapter 2. Take at least one scoop of Skinny Chick! Super Whey Protein a day in a shake; taking two to three scoops a day is better. You may also double up your scoop of whey protein in one shake if you are interested in building muscle. The scoop for measuring a serving is provided inside the container.

Skinny Chick! Calcium Magnesium

As you know from reading Chapter 3, you will be dumping minerals, including magnesium, so this one is also a must. My Skinny Chick! Calcium Magnesium supplement can be found in my online store on Amazon.com. Take four a day with food. Some people report that these supplements make them very relaxed or even sleepy (this would be caused by the magnesium) so it may be a good idea to take this supplement at dinner.

Potassium

In the first two weeks when your body is dumping potassium, as explained in Chapter 3, you need to take extra so you don't get leg cramps, dizziness, and low blood pressure. I have chosen Now brand Potassium Citrate 99mg to use with my program. Initially you will take three capsules, three times a day starting on day one through week two. At week three, you can cut down to three capsules a day unless cutting back causes leg cramps (which means your body is still dumping potassium at an accelerated rate). If you get leg cramps at any time, promptly take three to five Now brand Potassium Citrate 99mg supplements along with a salt shot and at least eight ounces of water and they should go away in thirty to forty-five minutes. If they do not, repeat the process until they do. For most people, one cycle of this will get rid of the leg cramps. This trick also works if you feel dizzy upon standing, which can mean your blood pressure is a little low. It can also do wonders for exhaustion in the first three days when your body is transitioning into ketosis.

I specifically picked potassium citrate for the potassium formula to use with my program because it can help with your kidney function. Do not worry about taking it as often as you feel you need it the first week when you may get leg cramps and need extra. Stick to the three capsules, three times a day dosage initially unless you need more. It would be very difficult to overdose on it, especially when your body will be dumping potassium at an accelerated rate.

Salt Shots

Your body will dump sodium while on protocol. Do a salt shot with real sea salt as needed and at least three times a day the first week along with your potassium supplement. Put ½– 1 tsp and up to 1½ tsp of Real Salt brand salt in your hand, put it in your mouth, and swallow it with at least eight ounces of water. If you get enough sodium from your food, you may not need to do salt shots beyond the first week. Salt vegetables liberally with the Real Salt brand sea salt or with any quality brand that contains all of the minerals in it.

Sodium has received a bad rap due to all of the highly processed food with high sodium content. However, sodium is an essential mineral. Most of the salt sold today is simply the wrong kind of salt. If the salt you are eating is pure white, it is most likely unhealthy and unfit for consumption. There are a few places in the world where you can get very pure sea salt that is pure white and it will be very expensive. Most healthy salt will contain brown "flecks" in it or color aside from just white. This means that the minerals are still intact and have not been processed out. As mentioned above, the brand Real Salt makes a very high quality, minimally processed and healthy salt. It is also very affordable. I get mine at Sprout's, but you can also get it on Amazon.com by searching Real Salt.

I have the occasional client who cannot tolerate doing the salt shots. For these clients, I suggest they purchase empty supplement capsules, which you can get at most health food stores and are inexpensive. They find filling up the capsules with their sea salt and swallowing them with their water and potassium supplement much more tolerable.

Recommended Supplements

There are too many supplements that I would love to mention in this book but I can't get into every supplement that I ever recommend and love. Throughout the book, however, I have recommended supplements aside from the required supplements to enhance your results. Here are the instructions on taking these as well as where to get them.

Skinny Chick! Thermo

Skinny Chick! Thermo is an excellent thermogenic, which again is a supplement that can accelerate your body's fat burning capacity. This blend contains a lot of fat burning and energy enhancing natural ingredients. It does contain caffeine, and I do not recommend it for nursing mothers, pregnant women, or anybody who has heart issues of any kind. The dosage is one tablet up to two times a day before breakfast and lunch but I would consider cutting one tablet in half the first two doses so you can see how you respond. This is a pretty powerful supplement that most people handle well and love. It can be too strong for some however so start out slow and allow your body to adjust if you need to. This supplement also acts as an excellent appetite suppressant. If you take it after 3:00, it will very likely keep you awake at night.

Skinny Chick! EPA/DHA

I am a big proponent of getting plenty of healthy fat in one's diet. One great way to help boost that goal is to supplement with a very good EPA/DHA Omega 3 supplement. This is a super food supplement and the effect that taking a good one can have on your health may surprise you. EPA and DHA are both types of Omega 3 fatty acids. One health benefit that most people have heard about is that Omega 3s can reduce your LDL cholesterol levels (bad cholesterol, I remember this by thinking lousy cholesterol) and boost your HDL cholesterol levels (good cholesterol that helps keep the LDL cholesterol at a healthy level. I remember this by remembering happy cholesterol). But this is just one of the many amazing things this supplement can do for your health. It has also been shown to boost brain function and is in fact essential for brain health. One of my favorite benefits is its ability to lower inflammation of all kinds anywhere in the body. This means that it can help with any kind of autoimmune disorder or any other disease that is linked to chronic inflammation, which I can't come close to covering in this little book. Skinny Chick! EPA/DHA, which is an excellent source of Omega 3 and a reasonably priced option, can be found in my online store at Amazon.com.

Skinny Chick! Bloat Eraser

As I have mentioned, a common complaint can be water retention while doing longer periods of the Skinny Chick! Rapid Fat Loss Protocol. Let's be honest, this is just a common complaint for women in general. The first thing to do to alleviate the bloating is to ensure you are drinking enough water. Your body will conserve water by retaining it if you are not consuming enough water. You also have the option of just dealing with the water retention and waiting for it to pass. I do find that this can lead to people getting discouraged, as it not only will make the numbers on the scale go up, it will also make you feel "fluffier" around the middle. It also tends to skew your fat percentage readings if you take my advice and purchase a scale that tells you your fat percentage.

Another option is to take a supplement to take the bloating away, such as Skinny Chick! Bloat Eraser, which is gentle enough to take on a regular basis without putting strain on your kidneys, as many over the counter diuretics can. It also has ingredients that can aid in kidney and liver detoxification. While taking any kind of diuretic, ensure that you drink plenty of water and consider adding an electrolyte, such as Emergen-C brand Electro Mix, if you are going to take it on a regular basis so that you will not disrupt your electrolyte balance.

Emergen-C Electro Mix

I have mentioned this supplement in a few places throughout this book. It is basically just a tasty and sugar free way to make a sports drink that will give you some of the electrolytes you need. My husband and I are addicted to this and always have it around the house. It is a nice thing to have to flavor your water with lemon-lime while on protocol or anytime. We get ours at Whole Foods, Sprouts, or on Amazon.com.

Green Vibrance

I got into the details of Green Vibrance in Chapter 4 so I won't get into them again here. It is my favorite super food supplement and the least expensive place to purchase it is Amazon.com

Probiotics

Probiotics are a supplement I think everybody should consider taking for their overall health and well-being. All the benefits of taking a probiotic are beyond the scope of this book but as I mentioned in Chapter 3, our guts should have around 80–85% good bacteria and 15–20% bad bacteria.

Because of the fact that most people have taken multiple rounds of antibiotics in their lifetime and that a lot of things aside from the added antibiotics in our food can kill off the good bacteria in our gut, most people do not have the correct ratio. There are too many good ones on the market to list here, but my favorite one to recommend and the one I use personally is New Chapter brand Primal Defense Ultra.

pH Drops

There are also a lot of alkalizing pH drops on the market: the two I have used and recommend to my clients are Natural Balance brand AlkaMax Alkaline Booster, which can be purchased on Amazon.com, and pH ion Balance brand Booster drops that can be purchased at most health food stores and at Amazon.com. These are great products to help you get through plateaus faster. If you do decide to take these, make sure you ease into them slowly. Taking them at full dosage too quickly can bring on an intense Herxheimer's Reaction. This is because some pathogens have a hard time surviving in an alkaline environment and when you get your acidity under control they will die off rapidly.

Stevia

Stevia is a wonderful alternative to sugar as it does not cause an insulin spike and it does not add calories. Stevia is an herb that has a very good safety profile with no ill health effects known. The only issue with stevia is it can sometimes be very bitter or can just taste off. Whole Foods 365 brand stevia is the best I have personally found. It comes in vanilla or regular flavored and can be purchased in packets or in a bottle. It takes very little stevia to sweeten whatever you put it in as it is much sweeter than sugar. It is well worth the effort to find a stevia that you like the flavor of, especially if you would like to continue sweetening things without the detrimental effects of sugar and artificial sweeteners.

Smooth Move

Smooth move comes in tea or capsule form. I have found the tea at several grocery stores and Walgreens but I have only found the capsules at Amazon.com. These are fairly strong laxatives and should only be used as needed so that you don't gain dependency on them. I prefer the tea when I use it so that I can make it stronger or weaker as needed according to how long it is steeped.

Chapter 9
Skinny Chick!
Rapid Fat Loss Recipes

Cucumber Dressing

2 large chopped cucumbers

1–2 garlic cloves (optional)

4 tbsp. olive or grapeseed oil

¼ cup Vegenaise

Sea salt to taste

Puree cucumbers and olive or grapeseed oil in blender

Add Vegenaise to cucumber puree and add sea salt to taste

Creamy, Spicy Mustard Dressing

One part spicy brown mustard, one part Vegenaise

Dipping Sauce for Meat

Mix Vegenaise with horseradish, low carb ketchup or mustard

Cocktail Sauce

Low carb ketchup mixed with horseradish to taste

Ranch, Dill or Onion Dip

Simply Organic Ranch, Dill or Onion dip mixes (found at Sprouts, some grocery stores and Whole Foods) mixed with Vegenaise

Meat "Breading"

Mix part Simply Organic Ranch, Dill, or Onion Dip with powdered parmesan cheese, dip meat in egg whites, and dip in mixture, pack extra on top. Searing both sides of meat in olive oil before baking will help make the "breading" crunchy. A small amount of almonds on top can also be added for more crunch

Deviled Eggs

Take one hard-boiled egg with approximately 1–1½ tsp. Vegenaise and mustard or a little horseradish if desired

Remove the yolk and mix it with the Vegenaise, add the mustard or horseradish to taste and put the mixture back in the egg. Sprinkle with a little cayenne or paprika

Basic Soup Recipe

Put your 2 cups of finely chopped, approved vegetables in a pot along with your 6-8 ounces of meat cut up. Add chicken, beef, or vegetable broth to taste, season with Mrs. Dash seasonings and sea salt to taste, cook until vegetables are to desired softness, enjoy (especially good with homemade chicken broth)

Cook approximately 6-8 ounces of turkey sausage. Chop 2 cups of zucchini (or any approved vegetable) and put in a pot, add fresh parsley, Tomato Basil Mrs. Dash brand seasoning, and sea salt to taste cook until vegetables are to desired softness, enjoy!

Pesto noodles

Prepare Miracle Noodles per package instructions. Add pesto to taste and a little bit of parmesan

Olive Oil and Parmesan Miracle Noodles

Prepare Miracle Noodles per package instructions. Add olive oil and parmesan plus some sea salt if desired

Stuffed Peppers or Mushrooms

Cook 1 pound of chicken or turkey sausage, add ¼–½ cup of grated parmesan, ¼–½ cup of diced mushrooms (if making it into stuffed mushrooms, skip the diced mushrooms), about 2 tbsp. of Vegenaise and a couple tsp of Mrs. Dash Onion Herb seasoning. Stuff either two green, gutted bell peppers or as many mushrooms as it takes and cook at 350 until pepper or mushrooms are soft. If there is any leftover meat, it can be put in the refrigerator to make a great addition to an omelet

Herb Infused Olive or Grapeseed Oil

Blend any herb with olive or grapeseed oil in blender (any excess can be stored in refrigerator). Leek, rosemary, cilantro, dill, and parsley are my favorites

Cauliflower with Leek and Parmesan

Chop and steam one whole head of cauliflower, add leek herb infusion to taste (test as you go, if it gets too strong you might not like it), add about 2 tbsp. Vegenaise, ¼ cup grated parmesan (the powdered stuff works best), and sea salt to taste. Double batches are recommended and can be put in the refrigerator. This recipe can also be good with the other flavors of herb infusions

Herb Infused Chicken or Turkey Burger

Blend ground turkey or chicken with an herb infused olive or grapeseed oil, blend to taste, sea salt to taste, and pan fry or grill (very good dipped in the Vegenaise and horseradish sauce)

Two to three Over Medium or Scrambled Eggs with leftover Cauliflower with Leek

Two to three over-medium or scrambled eggs over one serving of Cauliflower with Leek

Pumpkin Spice Greek Yogurt

Mix one serving of Chobani Unsweetened Greek Yogurt, with 1–2 tsp Bakto Pumpkin Pie flavoring, and Stevia and pumpkin pie spice to taste. This can be done with any of the Bakto flavorings, which again you can find on Amazon.com

Creamed Spinach

16 oz. frozen spinach cooked in pot, melt ¼ cup grated cheddar, ¼ cup grated parmesan, 2 tbsp. of half and half, sea salt to taste. This can't be an every night veggie as it has a little bit too much cheese to have often, stick to 1–2 times a week at most

Cauliflower Crust

2 eggs

1 head of cauliflower

¼ cup of olive oil

Seasonings to taste (depending on crust you are making, read more below)

Parmesan or Mozzarella Cheese, or both (optional)

¼ cup coconut or almond flour

Real Salt

Beat eggs in bowl until thoroughly beaten. Put raw cauliflower through food processor, do not puree but chop very, very small. Place around half of the finely chopped cauliflower in bowl with beaten egg (this will depend on how thick you want your crust to be as well as how big the head of cauliflower is). Add desired spices. For example, if I am making it into a pizza, I might put in Italian Seasoning. If I am making it into enchilada casserole, I might add in paprika and some chili powder. You may optionally add parmesan, mozzarella, or really any kind of cheese, as well as the coconut or almond flour (do not use the almond or coconut flour while on protocol) to make it stick together and take on more of a bread-like texture. Add a little bit of real sea salt, a couple teaspoons or so depending on taste. Add olive oil until it is sticking together pretty well. Put olive oil in the bottom of a cooking pan. I find glass, Pyrex type cooking pans to work the best. Press the crust down evenly in the pan on top of the olive oil (heat the olive oil in the oven before you place the cauliflower on top for a crispier crust bottom). Take some paper towel and remove as much moisture from the mixture as possible. Cook in a 400 degree oven until it is lightly browned to very browned on top (you will figure out your preference) around 30–40 minutes

*With this crust, you will have many options for good casseroles without all of the carbohydrates of bread crusts and with the benefit of adding extra veggies to whatever you are making. Following are some ideas of how I use the crust. Always prepare and then cook the cauliflower crust and then add on and heat up the toppings, otherwise your crust will be soggy. Also pre-sauté or steam any veggie you are putting on top, otherwise they will not cook all the way through. Unless you like the particular veggie crispy, for example, I do not pre-cook the bell peppers in my pizza or enchilada recipe, as I like them more crispy and fresh. It all depends on your preference.

Quiche with Cauliflower Crust

Cook sausage, some bell peppers, onions, and mushrooms (or whatever you like in your quiche), mix together, and then spread on top of cauliflower crust. Beat enough eggs to cover the top of the casserole, add some cheese if wanted, along with some real sea salt and pour on top of the mixture. Cook at 350 degrees until done all the way through about 30–45 minutes (keep an eye on it, as it will depend on your oven).

Pizza with Cauliflower Crust

Put pizza sauce on top of cooked cauliflower crust (very lightly, watch your carbs); add desired pizza toppings, pop back in 400 degree oven until toppings are melted and to your desired brownness.

Enchilada Casserole with Cauliflower Crust

Spread enchilada sauce over cooked cauliflower crust (very lightly watch your carbs); top it with cooked chicken or beef with the seasonings already cooked in (you can buy packets of enchilada or taco seasoning at the store that work great), spread cooked or raw bell peppers, chives, and any other toppings desired on top of this, and sprinkle a little bit of cheese on top. Cook at 400 degrees until it is all melted and to your desired brownness. Serve with sour cream, shredded lettuce, fresh cilantro, and guacamole

Cauliflower Cheesy Bread

Sprinkle a little bit of whatever kind of cheese you like over the top of the finished cauliflower crust and pop back in oven at 400 degrees until it is to your desired brownness. Serve with marinara sauce

Taco Salad

1 pound of ground beef

1 package of McCormick brand taco seasoning

Chopped chives

Chopped green peppers

Leafy lettuce

Cheddar or pepper jack cheese

Salsa

Daisy brand Light Sour Cream

Cook the taco meat and add the seasoning. Toss the veggies together; place the meat and cheese on top. Make the salad dressing out of the sour cream and salsa

Zucchini Casserole

3-4 large zucchinis chopped

Mushrooms chopped

10 ounces Ricotta cheese (the whole milk version, 2 g carbohydrates or under)

1 cup tomato sauce (canned marina sauce typically has the lowest carbohydrate content, 4g carbohydrate or under)

2 tbsp. Italian seasoning

1 tbsp. garlic powder or fresh garlic

1 tbsp. onion powder

8 oz. grated Italian cheese blend

½ cup powdered Parmesan

1-1 ½ pounds of sausage, cooked

Fresh, chopped parsley to taste (optional)

Mix all ingredients together (set some of the Italian Cheese Blend aside to put on top). Bake at 350 degrees until the zucchini is soft and the cheese on top is a little bit brown, about 45 minutes.

Whole Chicken with Veggies

Whole Chicken

Onion powder

Garlic powder

Sea salt

Olive oil

Fresh parsley

Green beans

Turnips

Take a whole chicken, wash it and place it in the middle of a large roasting pan. Add green beans and chopped up turnips around the chicken. With a basting brush, brush all veggies and the whole chicken with olive oil. Sprinkle all veggies and the chicken with onion powder and garlic powder as well as sea salt (and any other spices you want to add, get creative, I like it with just the onion and garlic powder with sea salt though), Place a handful of fresh parsley swigs inside the chicken (while <u>not</u> on protocol I also add chopped onions). Tie the legs together with thread (optional, I just do this to make it pretty when it comes out). Bake it in oven at 400 degrees for about 15 minutes to sear the chicken (searing is what keeps the juices inside the meat), then turn the oven down to 350 degrees. Baste the veggies and chicken with a basting brush about every 20-30 minutes until chicken is cooked to 165 degrees internally (you will need a meat thermometer, you can get these at any grocery or home goods store). When the chicken is cooked to 165 degrees internally, place it on top of the oven, baste it with the basting brush one more time, cover it with tin foil and then put a towel on top. Let it sit for 20 minutes (this allows the juices to redistribute and makes the chicken very moist and juicy), cut up and enjoy. You may need to add a little more sea salt to the veggies. The carcass can be boiled with fresh parsley and onion either in the crock-pot or on top of the stove to make a delicious chicken broth as a base for any soup recipe.

Mushroom Chicken and Sausage Casserole

3-4 cups of diced, cooked chicken

1 pound of cooked sausage

1 stock of celery finely chopped

Chopped mushrooms

4 ounces of ricotta cheese and 4 ounces of cream cheese (or all ricotta cheese)

Approximately 16 ounces or about a small head of cauliflower chopped and steamed

Grated cheddar or cheddar jack cheese

About 2 tsp of sea salt

2 tbsp. onion powder

1 tbsp. garlic powder or fresh garlic

Combine all ingredients and mix well (keep some of the grated cheese out to place on top), bake in 400 degree oven until the top is browned and it is heated all the way through, about 40 minutes

Low Carb Beef Stroganoff

1-1 ½ pounds cooked beef sirloin or tenderloin (ground hamburger works as well) cut into desired thickness, I like mine about ¼ an inch or so thick

2 tbsp. butter (optional)

2 tbsp. powdered onion

1 tbsp. powdered garlic (fresh can also be used if preferred, cook it with the mushrooms or meat)

Chopped mushrooms to taste

1 cup beef stock

½ cup coconut milk

1 tbsp. Dijon mustard (optional)

Cook the beef and set it aside. Cook chopped mushrooms with olive oil or coconut oil and set aside along with meat. Combine the butter, powdered onion, powdered garlic, 1 cup of beef stock, ½ cup coconut milk and Dijon mustard to same pan that the meat and mushrooms were cooked in and heat up. Add sour cream to hot yet not boiling beef stock and stir in. Add the cooked beef and mushrooms back to the pan, heat all of it up and allow it to thicken, add sea salt to taste.

Serve over miracle noodles, steamed cauliflower or steamed broccoli

Kale Chips

Cleaned, dried kale leaves removed from stems and torn into pieces

Olive oil

Sea salt

Coat Kale leaves with olive oil, do not drench them but make sure they are all evenly coated (make sure the kale is not wet from washing, this will make your chips soggy instead of crispy), spread evenly over a cookie sheet with parchment paper on top and sprinkle with sea salt to taste. Cook at 300 degrees for about 25 minutes depending on your oven rotating the cookie sheet once until kale chips are to desired crispiness. Allow them to cool for a few minutes

Eggcado (Avocado and Egg Bake)

Cut an avocado in half and remove the pit. Crack and place contents into each side of the avocado (some of the meat of the avocado may have to be removed to allow the entire egg to fit); sprinkle with sea salt to taste, jalapenos can be added on top if you would like a little spice. Cook at 425 degrees until the egg is all the way done, about 15 minutes. Add toppings if desired… hot sauce, a little bit of cooked bacon, chives and a little sour cream are all good choices or just eat it as is

Zucchini Ravioli

Zucchini

Olive Oil

Cooked Sausage

Cooked, Chopped mushrooms

Lowest Carbohydrate plain, canned tomato sauce you can find (4 g carbohydrates or less)

Italian Cheese

Italian Seasonings

Cut zucchini into thin slices and place on cooking sheet layered on top of each other in a cross shape, brush with olive oil. Combine cooked sausage, cooked mushrooms, a little bit of Italian cheese as well as Italian seasoning to taste. Put this mixture in the middle of each zucchini stack. Fold each of the four zucchini ends over the middle and secure them with a toothpick so they resemble a closed piece of ravioli. Cook in oven at 350 degrees until zucchini is to desired softness…about 15-20 minutes. Heat up the tomato sauce and add very sparingly to the top of the cooked zucchini ravioli

Turnip Fries

Thinly slice cleaned and dried turnips and space them evenly on cooking sheet with parchment paper or silicone on top. Brush them with olive oil with a basting brush and add sea salt to taste. Other spices can also be added, onion and garlic powder are both very good as are some of the Mrs. Dash brand seasonings. Bake at 425 degrees for about 30 minutes flipping once at about 15 minutes, turn the oven up to 450 and let them cook for an additional 15 minutes or so until they brown a little bit on top.

Parmesan Crisps

Place grated parmesan in little stacks on a parchment or silicone lined cooking sheet, bake at 400 degrees or until melted and a little browned and crispy.

Zucchini and Parmesan Chips

Place thinly sliced zucchini on either a silicone lined cooking sheet or a tin foil lined cooking sheet pre-brushed with olive oil, lightly brush zucchini with a small amount of olive oil, spread a little bit of parmesan on each zucchini slice and sprinkle with a little bit of sea salt. Broil on the top rack with the rack moved to the top of the oven until the cheese is a little browned and the zucchini is a little softened with crispy edges. Keep an eye on them while they cook so they do not burn, they should not take longer than about 10 minutes to cook.

Shake Recipes

Basic Shake Recipe

You will need a 20 oz. blender bottle, which can be purchased at most health food stores or at Amazon.com. Fill the blender bottle up halfway with unsweetened coconut milk (ensure it is unsweetened), put in one or two scoops of Skinny Chick! Super Whey Protein Mix in any of the three flavors (vanilla, chocolate and strawberry), add stevia if you would like, I find it too sweet this way. Fill the rest of the blender bottle up with either unsweetened vanilla, plain or chocolate almond milk (ensure the almond milk is also unsweetened)

Double Chocolate

All ingredients from basic shake recipe with unsweetened chocolate almond milk and chocolate Skinny Chick! Super Whey Protein Mix

1-1 ½ tsp. Bakto chocolate flavoring (optional)

Double Vanilla

All ingredients from basic shake recipe with unsweetened vanilla almond milk and vanilla Skinny Chick! Super Whey Protein Mix

1-1 ½ tsp. Bakto vanilla flavoring or vanilla extract (optional)

Pumpkin Spice

All ingredients from basic shake with unsweetened vanilla almond milk and vanilla Skinny Chick! Super Whey Protein Mix

1-1 ½ tsp. Bakto pumpkin pie flavoring

Cinnamon, cloves and nutmeg to taste

Pumpkin Spice Latte

All ingredients from pumpkin spice shake except for almond milk (unless instant coffee is used)

1 cup of hot or cold coffee instead of almond milk or add instant coffee to taste

1 tbsp. half and half (optional)

*Put all cold ingredients in, shake then add hot coffee and stir it, never shake hot ingredients in your blender bottle, it will blow out everywhere when you open it and burn you.

Mocha Latte

All ingredients for double chocolate shake except for almond milk (unless instant coffee is used)

1 cup of hot or cold coffee instead of almond milk or add instant coffee to taste

1 tbsp. half and half (optional)

*Put all cold ingredients in, shake then add hot coffee and stir it, never shake hot ingredients in your blender bottle, it will blow out everywhere when you open it and burn you.

Vanilla Latte

All ingredients from double vanilla shake except for almond milk (unless instant coffee is used)

1 cup of hot or cold coffee instead of almond milk or add instant coffee to taste

1 tbsp. half and half (optional)

*Put all cold ingredients in, shake then add hot coffee and stir it, never shake hot ingredients in your blender bottle, it will blow out everywhere when you open it and burn you.

Vanilla Spiced Chai Tea Latte

All ingredients for double vanilla shake except for almond milk

Steep two chai spice tea packs in 1 cup boiling water until strong, add to vanilla shake

*Put all cold ingredients in, shake then add hot tea and stir it, never shake hot ingredients in your blender bottle, it will blow out everywhere when you open it and burn you.

Coconut Chocolate

All ingredients for basic shake with unsweetened chocolate almond milk and chocolate Skinny Chick! Super Whey Protein Mix

1 tsp. Bakto coconut flavoring

Almond Joy

All ingredients for coconut chocolate shake

Add almond extract

Mango Strawberry

All ingredients for basic shake with plain or vanilla almond milk and strawberry Skinny Chick! Super Whey Protein Mix

1-1 ½ tsp. Bakto mango flavoring

Chocolate Covered Strawberry

All ingredients for basic shake with unsweetened chocolate almond milk and chocolate or strawberry Skinny Chick! Super Whey Protein Mix

1 tsp. Bakto strawberry flavoring

Dreamsicle

All ingredients from basic shake with unsweetened vanilla almond milk and vanilla Skinny Chick! Super Whey Protein Mix

1-1 ½ tsp. Bakto orange flavor

Caramel

All ingredients from basic shake with unsweetened vanilla almond milk and vanilla Skinny Chick! Super Whey Protein Mix

1-1 ½ tsp. Bakto caramel flavoring

* Ice and ½ a serving of Chobani brand unsweetened Greek yogurt can be added to any shake to make a smoothie. If ½ a serving of yogurt is put in the shake, only ½ a serving should be eaten for a snack that day.

Chapter 10
Self Love

I understand the self love and brain exercise stuff in this chapter does not appeal to everybody but the truth is that it works for many people, even for some of the people who don't think it will work for them in my little clinic. In many cases, the reason people can't lose weight or can't lose weight and keep it off begins in their mind and with their feelings and emotions toward themselves. I call it the inner abuser, and it may be afflicting you whether you realize it or not.

I will tell you a personal story of how powerful our minds and our emotions can be to our health and bodies. When I was in my early twenties, I was in an abusive relationship. I felt trapped and powerless to get out of it. As you know if you read the introduction, this was the time in my life when my health went into a rapid decline. It started with a diagnosis of gastritis, then I had gastritis and gall bladder disease, then it turned into all of those and Crohn's disease. Somewhere in the midst of all of these health issues and a whole host of others that continued to surface, I also developed an issue with my heart and chest. I could not really explain the problem to my doctors nor could they tell me what it was but I would get heart "flutters" and it pretty much always felt like I had an elephant sitting on my chest making breathing labored and difficult. In fairness to my doctors, they probably could have told me it was stress related had I told them the truth about what was going on at home but I told them that everything was fine and that I had nothing to be stressed out about. This was of course not true, but I don't think one needs to have experienced an abusive relationship to understand how stressful it can be or to have as many health issues as I did to understand how afraid I was that my life was over. I also really loved and needed my abuser, making it that much more hurtful and painful to me. I could not stand the thought of losing him and in a lot of ways; I blamed myself and thought I deserved it... typical of an abused person unfortunately.

To the outside world, we were a perfect couple. We were in love; we lived in a beautiful home in a nice neighborhood, and had a great group of friends. He was a "classic" abuser in the sense that he did not abuse me in front of others. To the contrary, he was usually quite doting and sweet to me around other people. He also could be so wonderful sometimes and in between "abusive times", he would profusely apologize and promise it would never happen again. He made me feel so loved when he was not abusing me. On top of the fact that he hid it... I hid it too. In part because I loved him and wanted to protect him and in part because I am a perfectionist and I want everything to be perfect and certainly to appear perfect (which of course is completely ridiculous and unattainable. I am still getting this life lesson down). What went on behind closed doors at our house was not pretty. I was embarrassed and did not want anybody to see or know about it. He did slip a few times, mostly in front of my mom and a couple friends but most people were completely clueless about the hell I lived in. So what did I do with all of that pain, stress, anxiety? I internalized it... I did not deal with it... I did not get it out of me... I pushed it way down and pretended it did not exist. I understand now what I did not understand then: all of that negative energy was wreaking havoc on my body and manifesting as disease (dis-ease).

I got to a point where I finally saw the light and understood that if I stayed with this abuser I would die... literally and figuratively. I got up the courage to leave him and I told him he had to leave our home. He did what he always did, he cried and promised to change, begged and told me he could not live without me because he loved me so much. I had accepted that it would never change and I had made up my mind even though it hurt. I told him it was over, I had purchased him a plane ticket home, and my dad was on his way so he needed to pack a suitcase and leave immediately. He did not know that I had also opened our big windows in the front of the house and had called the police; there was an officer outside listening in case this was to turn into a dangerous situation. He finally relented after a lot of trying every angle of breaking me down from sobbing to trying to convince me he was the only person that would ever love me (because I was unlovable to all but him), with some serious verbal abuse to back up his claims.

As he was packing, I was sitting in the front close to the windows and was having serious difficulty breathing. I felt the heart flutters coming on. He walked up to the stairs on the opposite side of the room, stopped, told me I had one more chance to change my mind and with me shaking my head 'No', left the house sobbing and heart broken. My heart was broken too, and I was definitely about to have a "flutter attack". I watched him drive down the street in front of our house until he turned the corner and disappeared. I was devastated. I knew my life would never be the same. My love was gone. I would have to move out of the gorgeous home I loved so much because I could not afford it on my own. At the same time, I instantly realized something, my little flutter attack had stopped in its tracks and I could breath as if there were no longer an elephant on my chest. I was stunned. I realized for the first time in months how nice it is to be able to breath. I never had those particular issues again. All the rest of my health issues started to clear up slowly as well.

It would take a lot more time to get past all my health issues and a complete one-eighty-degree turn in my lifestyle. However, after being told that I needed my colon and gall bladder removed and that I'd never ever have children (which I very dearly wanted someday). After almost dying of a drug reaction and losing all hope of ever living a happy and healthy life, simply leaving an abusive relationship had an instant positive effect on my body. I had already begun getting into nutrition and a healthier lifestyle before this epiphany and it had helped me. I believe it got me well enough to see the light and have the strength to leave the relationship. Months and months of all of my efforts to live a healthy lifestyle did not come close to the instant relief I felt when I knew at a deep level I would not be abused anymore.

This is but one example of many I could give you just as it pertains to my life of how important the mind is to our overall health. This story was too painful to share for a very long time. The only person I told any details to for many years was my mom. Now, I share this very personal story with you to help you see that if you don't get your mind healthy, you will have a difficult time getting your body healthy.

Think about the placebo effect. Think about when you got your heart broken and you felt physical pain in your heart. The mind-body connection is powerful. This is why I ask that you at least try to internalize what I am saying about the possible reasons your body is manifesting extra weight, which I consider "dis-ease". You are not just a body: you are a mind, a spirit, a soul. So it would make sense that if you have an issue with your weight and health, it is coming from something. What are you really carrying around in that weight? If you would not like to even begin to buy into any of that then you can skip the whole mind-body connection section and skip to the challenge at the end of the book. I advise against it though, as one thing I see over and over is the clients who are willing to do all the work necessary to change themselves and are not just looking for the shortcut get much better short term and long term results.

Do I think what you eat is important? Um... yeah!! I went back to school to become a nutritionist and you just read this whole book about my opinion on how we should eat to attain vibrant health! I obsessively study nutrition still to this day! However, I am a person first and I know that if my head is not right, I don't do right (or eat right!). So if you are interested in beginning to get to the source of the issues that are causing you to have a dis-ease then read on; if not, that's okay too. You know what resonates with you. I will tell you that although nutrition changed my life, I credit changing my thought patterns and learning to let go of all of the pain I have experienced for saving my life. The more I master the art of mastering my thoughts, the better my life gets. Please read on and give it a chance, even if you are not sure and skeptical. Try it... you have everything to gain and nothing to lose.

What is Eating You?

Quit being so hard on yourself... nobody and I mean nobody is perfect, we set up this crazy ideal in our society that people need to be absolutely perfect. Well guess what, we are enforcing this ideal with images of people that don't exist. Yes, there are beautiful people in these images, who are airbrushed, in perfect lighting, with perfect, professional hair and makeup. Those images are not of people who got up, rolled out of bed, and had a snapshot taken. These images take serious time, money, and effort.

I remember seeing an image of Cindy Crawford, who I considered to be the most beautiful woman ever when I was younger, and there was a side by side of a before she was photo shopped picture and an after photo shop picture. They took inches off her already beautiful thighs and waist and did a bunch of other airbrushing to her to "perfect" her image. It made me feel terrible about myself. If Cindy Crawford wasn't pretty enough, how would I ever be pretty enough? After I saw this image, I saw a quote of hers that made me love her: "I wish I got up looking like Cindy Crawford." That says it all doesn't it? Even the most beautiful people in the world are not beautiful enough. So we live in this society where we strive to look like people who can't even live up to their own images... do you see how insane this is? It is time to adopt a more healthy way of approaching ourselves, where we realize that we will never attain absolute perfection and that is okay. We should only strive to be the best we can be. Do not compare yourself to people who don't exist or to anybody for that matter.

The flip side of this crazy ideal we can't live up to is there is a constant barrage of powerful and often very misleading advertising for foods that are horrible for you. Most people have metabolic disorders after years of eating this horrible food that makes them constantly crave it, making this advertising even more effective. So all too often, we make excuses and justifications: this is all I have time for... I will stop eating this tomorrow... I just need one more "fix." How do you feel after you give in and eat this food that you know is packing more pounds on you? You feel terrible, right? You feel lethargic, gross, and mad at yourself for eating it and helpless to break the cycle.

My clients come to me to try to better themselves. I listen to them as they try to explain to me how guilty they feel for taking this time and spending this money just for them. I have heard it so many times, 'I am not vain... I just want to feel better... I just want to feel better about myself.' Do you think that taking care of yourself is vain? Whew, I am very vain indeed then! I see it a very different way. I see taking exemplary care of this one and only temple we have to live in, our body as a form of self-love and treating our body the opposite way, as self-punishment or even self-hatred and sometimes self-protection. I can't tell you how deeply it hurts me when I hear a person say, 'I hate my body' or 'I look terrible.' Would you ever say such a thing to another human being? Probably not, but here you are saying this to yourself and worse, much worse. You are abusing yourself and beating yourself down! Of course you don't have the motivation to want to fix it; you don't love yourself enough to leave the abuser... that's right, you are the abuser. Would you not call it abuse to say to somebody you are ugly... you are fat? Do you say that to yourself? To deal with the pain, do you stuff it down with food, alcohol, etc.? This is making the problem worse and worse by setting your body up to crave these things through body chemistry and nutritional deficiencies. You are setting your body up through emotional turmoil and unhealthy lifestyle habits for disease, excess weight, and ultimately, the inability to lose it. Then hating what you see in the mirror and abusing yourself more. For a lot of people, it is a never-ending cycle.

So how do you deal with this? You look for the magic pill, the magic diet; the thing that you just know will finally make you lose this weight so you can finally love yourself! Of course, this fad stuff doesn't work or it does, but only until you go back to your old ways and gain it all back plus some. Some fads are even dangerous! Rinse and repeat... do I have that right? Of course I do... that is most likely why you are reading my book, correct?

In my experience, there is another reason that people do not succeed in getting to their best selves: self-protection. They are afraid of the attention that comes with attaining your best self. Perhaps somebody has treated you badly, done or said horrible things to you, and now you are afraid of any kind of attention? Maybe you just try to be invisible? Some of the attention you will get by getting your body where you want it is very positive; some of it unfortunately can be negative. I think some are afraid that when they get to their goal, people will reject their new lifestyle, accuse them of having an eating disorder, or think the things they are doing are ridiculous.

I have had many clients who were uncomfortable at first with all the attention they got from losing the weight and from everybody saying how amazing they looked… they got over it! Look, there will always be those people in the world, the ones who want to hold you back and keep you unhealthy and not your best self, just like them; people who are so busy being jealous of your accomplishments that they can't be happy for you. You have to decide to rise above them. I know that sounds harsh but I also know that you have to decide to tune the naysayers out if you want to succeed. Do you think for one second that there were not people who disagreed with me, didn't support me, and thought I was insane for attempting this radical shift in my lifestyle in lieu of just listening to my doctors and getting organs removed? There were too many naysayers to count! I listened to the voice inside me and tuned all the rest out for a little while. It got lonely at times but I personally could not fathom where I would be if I had not done that. I am glad I chose to love, honor, and listen to myself. I am glad I did the work to change my life for the better in every way. Looking back nothing has ever been so worth it.

Of course, it is not this dramatic for everybody is it. Some people just have bad habits, food or alcohol addictions, along with the body imbalances to keep them craving bad things. Some just have not found the right thing for their body. Some people only lack the motivation to do something about it. So what creates motivation? Success!! I know, I know, that makes no sense… you have to have the motivation to do it to get to the success part. So again, it all boils down to self-love. Do I love myself enough to change my ways and get my body, energy levels, and health to where I want it to be? Do I love myself enough to ignore the people who say I can't or shouldn't do it and rise above them? You have to get to that to get to the success part. I will say this: a lot of my clients have tried so many things with little or no success. These clients are amazed and delighted with how well this system works for them and they end up addicted to it! It is so much easier to stick to a program when you get results, and a healthy lifestyle is not such a bad thing to be addicted to! Don't let anybody tell you different. This is your life!

The good thing about this plan is it yields fast results when you do it right, which for many people keeps them very motivated indeed. Then when you follow it up with the healthy lifestyle and maintenance plan, you get to keep enhancing your results. People who get to this level of fit and healthy rarely go back because if feels really good! You have energy, stamina, and you feel good about how you look. If this program is done correctly, you will also stop having the horrible cravings that have plagued you in the past. Having been unbelievably unhealthy in my early twenties and now in my mid-thirties being the healthiest I have ever been, I can tell you hands down, I pick my body now over any food, beverage, or anything else because it just is not worth it. I also pick this body over the body I had in my twenties! How many people can say that? I am in great shape and it is now effortless… go figure! Being healthy, re-teaching yourself to care and think about what you put in your body… that is worth it. Rearranging your body chemistry so all those cravings that are so hard to shake leave you for good… worth it! Having mental clarity, energy, stamina to power through your day; trying on cute clothing and loving what you see in the mirror… totally worth it! I hate to break it to you though; you will have to do the work to get there. The following quote encompasses the path to real health…

"The elevator to success is out of order; you will have to take the stairs…
one step at a time."

Joe Girard

If you do this program to the letter, it will no longer be a struggle, you will eventually not crave sugar anymore and you will start to feel amazing and in control of your body. Who knows what other areas of your life will open up! So please at least give the following brain exercises a chance before you begin your weight loss program. They don't take a lot of time and they just may help you set your sight on success.

"We cannot become what we want to be by remaining who we are."

Max DePree

How Does Being Unhealthy Restrict You?

Grab a piece of paper or start a journal, clear your mind and fill out the following questions honestly and with the first answer that comes to your mind.

1. Can you buy and wear the clothing that you want to and feel comfortable in it?

Yes____ No____

2. Do you buy the clothing that you can tolerate wearing for your body type or to "camouflage" your problem areas?

Yes____ No____

3. What thoughts come to you when you look in the mirror? Be honest.

_____

_____

_____

_____

_____

_____

_____

4. Is there an activity you can't do because of your health status or weight that you would like to do? What are those activities?

_____

_____

_____

_____

_____

5. Do you have health issues? This includes not being in shape the way you want to be in.

Yes____ No____

6. How do these issues restrict you?

_____

_____

_____

_____

_____

_____

_____

"Many find eating healthy food and living a healthy lifestyle restrictive. How much more restricted are you if you can't wear the clothing you want to wear, can't participate in the activities you want to participate in, and don't feel good or have any energy? How restricted will you be when your unhealthy lifestyle catches up to you and you end up with a serious disease? Having a healthy lifestyle is the opposite of restrictive, it is empowering. It is never too late to be the person you want to be."

Robin Webb

How Becoming Healthy Will Free You

When it comes down to it, only you can decide to take charge of your health and body. Most people are acutely aware of how important a healthy lifestyle is. They just can't seem to get motivated to make the change. There are things that can help on the inevitable weak willed days however. Let's start with the questions we answered before, with a more positive spin...

7. Can you imagine yourself being as healthy as you want to be and being at the fitness level you want to be at? If not, can you at least attempt to picture it?

Yes____ No_____

8. What clothing will you purchase when you get to your goal?

_____

_____

_____

_____

_____

_____

9. What thoughts would you like to come to your mind when you look in the mirror?

_____

_____

_____

10. What activities will you be partaking in when you hit your health and fitness goals?

_____

_____

_____

11. What health issues are you going to get rid of in the near future?

_____

_____

_____

12. What restrictions will you be leaving behind when you get where you want to be?

_____

_____

_____

13. What is your X factor? What is driving you to meet your goal?

_____

_____

_____

14. Are you willing to change your ways so you can get the body you want?

Yes_____   No_____

15. Are you willing to stick with this until you hit your goal?

Yes_____   No_____

Questions 1–6 focus on what you can't do; questions 7–15 focus on what you can do. Your mental state is as important as your physical state when it comes to health. Too many people grossly underestimate the power of the mind. Try to edge negative self-talk out of your mind. Try to replace thoughts like, I can't do this; I am not good enough; I am not strong enough to go through with this, by pushing the delete button when these thoughts pop up and replacing them with thoughts like: I will do this! I am good enough! I am strong enough and I will see this through! Focus on what you want as opposed to what you don't want. Write down some affirmations below. Popular ones are; I Love and Accept Myself (coined by Louise Hay) and You Are Perfect Just the Way You Are. Only you know your personal problems with yourself.

Read these as often as you need to and at least two times a day. Really feel what you are saying. Look at yourself in the mirror while you say them. It is important to decide to love and accept yourself now and not have the attitude of 'I will love myself when I get to my goal.' As I stated above, if you can't start cultivating self-love now and you keep abusing yourself, you will be much less likely to love yourself enough to free yourself of this weight and your inner abuser. Tell yourself how proud you are that you are taking charge of this issue once and for all! I remember the first time I tried to look in the mirror and tell myself 'I love you.' It made me giggle and then it made me sad because I did not mean it... at all. Work on this, you will take better care of yourself if you learn to love and respect yourself now. You will be better and more loving in every area of your life (partner, parent, sister, brother, friend, etc.), if you learn to love and respect yourself first.

Another good tool for creating a positive self-image is visualization. Visualize yourself in the clothing you want to wear and the shape and the health state you want to be in. Go back to question number 7; if you can't see yourself where you want to be, you aren't as likely to be able to get there. Start visualizing yourself where you want to be until you believe you can get there. This will become easier when you start seeing results and get to the realization that this does work. It may feel unnatural at first if you can't see yourself getting where you want to be. You must keep working on seeing it though. Knowing within you that you can achieve your goal is as important as following the program correctly. Imagine and feel how good it would feel to get to your goal and hold onto that feeling.

I guess I am saying the most important tip anybody can give you is... love yourself. Eating very unhealthy food and not taking care of oneself can be viewed as punishment to oneself. So what are you punishing yourself for? I promise you don't deserve it. Forgive yourself! On the other hand, taking care of yourself can be viewed as loving yourself. Eating healthy, giving your body enough rest, exercise, sunshine, and joy is part of the pursuit of happiness we are all living. What is the point to any of it if we are miserable, unhealthy, and unable to do and enjoy the things we want to do and enjoy? Things are beautiful when you love them, and you are no different. Stop picking out your flaws and emphasize the positive things about yourself... I guarantee you have a lot of them. We all have flaws but I promise you that yours are much more evident to you than anybody else. Our relationship with ourselves may arguably be the most difficult relationship we will ever have. Treat <u>yourself</u> the way you want to be treated! You are one of a kind; really, there is nobody like you anywhere! Instead of disliking yourself for what you are not, love and accept yourself for all of the amazing things that you are! Love yourself as if your life depends on it, because it does. I am not asking you to accept your weight that you want to lose... you can lose it. I am asking you to give yourself a big pat on the back and be very proud of yourself for doing something about it and look forward to the day when it is no longer an issue. I have never had a client sit across my desk and been able to agree with them that they are unworthy and not beautiful the way they are. I always see the beauty that they don't see. I know you have it too. Focus on becoming a better version of yourself. You are already perfect and the only one of your kind. I guarantee if I could spend some time with you, I could pick out five beautiful things about you in under a minute! It is not difficult to do at all, until it comes to picking them out while we are looking in the mirror.

Write Down at least Five Amazing things about you... I know for a fact there are many more than five things!

_____

_____

_____

_____

_____

_____

_____

From now on, focus on the amazing things about yourself. Forget that other stuff in the past, it doesn't matter now. If you dwell on the past, you cripple the now. Every time one of those nagging, negative, nasty thoughts about yourself or somebody else pops in your head, close your eyes, put it in a balloon, and release it or simply push the delete button then allow a positive thought. You will eventually have more and more positive thoughts. Positive thinking is so important to becoming healthy and to being happy. Think a negative thought... how do you feel? Weighed down... not good... low? Now think a positive thought... how do you feel? Uplifted... re-motivated... happy... good? Start learning to be a glass half-full kind of person. It will change your life. When thinking a negative thing about myself or another person, I find myself thinking 'That is not nice!' I then force myself to pick out something good and positive about myself or the other person. I do understand that it is not easy to think nice things about all people, trust me, I really do. Remember though, these ugly thoughts and feelings ever so slowly poison you, so start edging them out starting now.

Don't see changing your lifestyle as a burdensome thing that you have to endure to get to your goal. Think of changing your lifestyle as the wonderful things you get to do to put yourself in control of your weight and health. A way to free yourself from a body that does not support you and you don't want to look at yourself in the mirror in. A simple shift in how you perceive things. Turning something into a joyful choice you have control over as opposed to a burdensome task you must endure can make all the difference in your ability to follow through. Keep your eye on the prize. As you go along your path, the temptation to go back gets less and less. You just have to take that first step, then the next, then the next.

"Whether you think you can or think you can't, you are right."

Henry Ford

Another powerful tool for getting your mind detoxed is practicing forgiveness. People almost always give me a perplexed look when I say this. Forgiveness is very important for healing though. Holding onto things that you can't forgive yourself or others for will hinder your results.

Write down the things you need to forgive yourself for, including all the mean and abusive things you have said to yourself (get another piece of paper if you need to, I know I did).

_____

_____

_____

_____

_____

_____

_____

_____

_____

_____

_____

_____

_____

Now look in the mirror and tell yourself you forgive yourself for all of the above things. Say it over and over until you mean it. Take a deep breath and imagine each thing as a balloon that you let go and watch sail away. Do this as many times as you need to.

I am going to ask you to forgive anybody else who has wronged you too. Why do we need to forgive others? We don't forgive others for their sake, we forgive others for ourselves. *"Holding onto anger is like drinking poison and expecting the other person to die"* (unknown author) Pretty powerful right? What is your anger doing to the person you are angry at? Nothing… it is eating you up and not affecting them. Put these in a balloon in your mind and watch them float away too. Another thing I do with people who I have to cut out (such as the inner-abuser) is walk up to the edge of a foggy lake with them, watch them get on a boat, stand on the bank, and push them off into the water. I wave goodbye, as I watch them float away into the fog. I send them light and love and I tell them I will try to remember the good things about them and forget the bad things, and I let them go. I realize how cheesy this sounds but try it, it is freeing. I still have to re-do these steps above from time to time. Forgive yourself and forgive others. Do not say unacceptable behavior is okay, do not permit the behavior to continue but forgive what is in the past and let it go. Holding onto it will poison you.

Write down the things you need to forgive others for (again get another page if you need to, I know I did)

_____

_____

_____

_____

_____

_____

_____

_____

_____

_____

_____

_____

"Whatever it is, just let it go,
it is not worth it."

Michael Bernard Beckwith

Now that you have forgiven yourself and others (or are at least working on it), please take the time to write out this contract to yourself. This is another tool you can download with the free downloads at skinnychickweightloss.com if you would like a contract to yourself in a printable version. This is a great tool to put on your fridge as a reminder in weak moments.

I_____ (your name) have allowed unhealthy and destructive habits to overtake my life. I hereby commit to love myself enough to take care of this beautiful temple (my body) that is the only home I have to live in. I have the power to undo these unhealthy habits and replace them with new and healthy habits and that is just what I am going to do. I am special and unique, there is nobody anywhere quite like me. I have these beautiful traits (go back to the five things you love about yourself and insert them here)

_____

_____

_____

_____

_____

_____

and I love that about myself. I fill myself with love and gratitude for this big opportunity to learn how to treat my body with the love and respect it deserves. I am willing to change. I love myself enough to give my body what it needs to heal and repair so that I may be free of these bad habits forever. I release the need to abuse myself any longer. I cut the ethereal cord of anybody who wants to hold me back from being the best person I can be, including the inner abuser that I will no longer feed. I forgive myself for setting up these patterns but I will no longer allow these patterns to remain starting _____ (your starting date), I will start my life anew and follow through with this commitment to myself. This contract is binding. If I get knocked off of my healthy path for whatever reason, I will not beat myself up about it for I am only human. I will pick myself up, dust myself off, and continue right back on my path. I will do this as many times as I need to because I am worth it! I release all of the pain from the past that has caused me to stuff my feelings down. I release anything and anybody that no longer serves me.

Furthermore, I promise myself to (Fill in any other thing you want to add to better yourself)

_____

_____

_____

_____

_____

_____

_____

_____

_____

_____

Your Signature

_____

With the contract, find a quiet spot where you can spend ten to twenty minutes focusing on visualizing your goals. Close your eyes and take five deep breaths, feel your muscles relaxing. Fill yourself up with light and love by visualizing a light coming through the top of your head and filling you up. Let the light fill every corner in you that still thinks you can't do it or still wants to say or do harmful things to you. Let the light chase these things out through the top of your head. Let all the areas that you are clearing the negativity from fill with love for yourself and gratitude that you do have a way out of where you don't want to be. Open your eyes and read your contract to yourself, feel the words you are saying, let them sink in. Close your eyes again and feel your resolve to lovingly free yourself from that which no longer serves you. Do this exercise as often as you need. If you can do it once or twice every day, that is ideal. Do it as often as you want to or need to.

You and only you have the power to free yourself from this. Stop using 'I don't know how' as an excuse. You now have a real, tangible way that does work... what will you do with it? If you have not picked it up already, I am a tad passionate about teaching people how to better themselves. I actually consider all of the very difficult things I have been through with my health and just in life in general to be a blessing. If I had never been that low, I would never have had to find my way out of it and I would never have learned the absolute joy that comes with lighting the way for others. I used to really and truly hate myself. I was never enough, and it seemed to make me draw people who further drained me into my life. Now I can wholeheartedly say that I love and respect myself in a non-egotistical or self-centered but healthy and good way. My capacity to love others, the way I see the world, my capacity for compassion and so much more changed so beautifully and drastically when I learned this key tool for health and wellness. Now I am so full of love and life that I am able to overflow it to others. My life has opened up so much just from this one simple, yet unbelievably difficult thing called loving myself. Start working on it today and watch your world change for the better in every way.

One big challenge you will have with following a new diet is this: our culture revolves around food, way too much in my opinion. Think about this, what do you do when you want to celebrate? You probably reach for food, alcohol, or both. What do you do when you feel bad about something? You probably reach for food, alcohol, or both. I am not saying stop enjoying food. I LOVE food and wine by the way. It is not all there is though. Try to find other ways to reward and nurture yourself. I love a good book, a good talk with somebody I love, a massage, getting my nails done, a cute new outfit or shoes. You may love a nice bath, a walk, cuddling with your kids or pets... whatever it may be, figure out what it is that makes you happy. Teach yourself to reach for that instead of food when you want to celebrate or nurture yourself. Don't expect yourself to be perfect all the time, expect to mess up and fall off your chosen path. Just hop right back on, no worries. I also really encourage people to take it easy with this and not become obsessed about everything you put in your mouth. It took a long time to get to your current health and weight status... allow some time to undo it. I get that once you decide you want something a certain way you want it now. Trust me, I understand that a lot. Getting yourself back to a healthy state and the weight you want to be is not going to happen overnight. It will take time and commitment... you are worth it.

Three times I bow

Letting go, letting be

I honor the core

I set myself free

The Challenge

You have had a great deal of information put into your head, and I hope you have found it interesting and helpful. Now what will you do with it? I would like to propose a challenge. Do everything I have laid out in this book for one whole month. Do the Skinny Chick! Rapid Fat Loss Protocol for three weeks straight and consider that your boot camp. For the other week in your one-month challenge, eat low on the glycemic index and stick to eating close to protocol, only with more carbohydrates added in from vegetables not included on protocol and some fruit. Take pictures of yourself before you start and measure your loss as I have it laid out in Chapter 6 so you can watch yourself melt. Completely invest yourself to one whole month of working hard to get results with no cheating. When you see the results you can get from just one month of this, you will be hooked. Remember earlier when I said that results give the best motivation? Start getting results. The more results you get, the more motivated you will be to continue. Get yourself addicted to health.

This concludes my labor of love. Please let me finish by saying you can do this! Please allow this to change your life for the better, as it has for so many of my clients. I do offer guided programs with access to me to answer your questions, look over your food journal weekly (to make sure you are doing it correctly), as well as bi-weekly group webinars or one-on-one consultations to help keep you motivated and on track. There is also just so much more to this, more than I could ever put in one book. I highly encourage you to be part of the conversation by joining the Skinny Chick! Community on facebook for help and support from your peers as well as additional tips and resources. Just search <u>Skinny Chick! Community</u> on facebook and join!

Please visit my health and wellness clinic, Complete Weight Loss and Wellness at <u>www.completeweightlossandwellness.com</u> for more information and to sign up for my guided programs. Also remember that you can go to <u>skinnychickweightloss.com</u> to download helpful tools and resources, such as a printable version of the Skinny Chick! Rapid Fat Loss Protocol, measurement chart, weekly food log, glycemic index food chart, and a contract to yourself for when you need a reminder of why you have committed yourself to this program. I will also send you a shopping list to bring with you to the store when you get started on the Skinny Chick! Rapid Fat Loss Protocol and a PDF about how to cook and shop for healthy, yet delicious food as well as how to read nutrition labels.

I wish you vibrant health, self love, and joy for the rest of your days. I hope you have enjoyed reading Skinny Chick! as much as I enjoyed writing it.

-Robin Webb

"The tragedy of life is not that it ends so soon, but that we wait so long to begin it."

C.W. Lewis